THE MIND DIET COOKBOOK

A Complete Cookbook with 140 Recipes to manage Alzheimer's, Dementia and improve your brain's health Including a 10-Day Meal Plan

Zera wright

© 2023 by Zera Wright

All rights reserved. No part of this book may be reproduced or transmitted in any form or by any means, electronic or mechanical, including photocopying, recording, or by any information storage and retrieval system, without permission in writing from the publisher.

The recipes and information contained in this book are for educational and informational purposes only, and are not intended as medical advice or a substitute for professional medical care. The author and publisher are not responsible for any adverse effects or consequences that may result from the use of the information or recipes in this book.

While the author and publisher have made every effort to ensure that the information in this book is accurate and up-to-date, they make no representations or warranties of any kind, express or implied, about the completeness, accuracy, reliability, suitability, or availability with respect to the information or recipes contained in this book for any purpose. Any reliance you place on such information is therefore strictly at your own risk.

DEDICATION

To my family and friends,

I want to thank you all for helping me realize my dream of becoming an author. Without your encouragement and support, this book would not have been possible. You have all been my biggest cheerleaders and have been there for me every step of the way. From brainstorming ideas, to helping me with the editing process, to promoting the book, you have been there every step of the way.

I am so grateful for all the love and support you have given me over the years. Your kind words and encouragement have meant the world to me.

This book is dedicated to every individual who has had to struggle with weight issues and is looking for a healthier lifestyle. I hope that this book will provide the information and support they need to make a successful transition to a healthier lifestyle.

Thank you again for your never-ending support and love.

Sincerely,

Henrietta Conner, Author of The Complete Gastric Sleeve Bariatric Cookbook

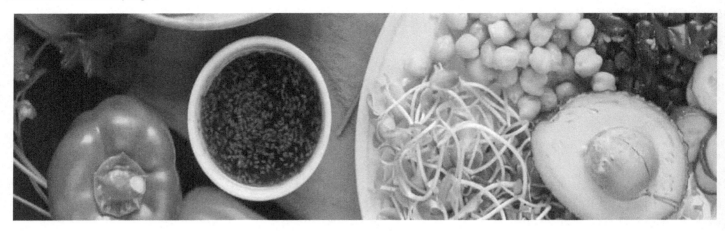

Table of Contents

About the Writer _____ 10

INTRODUCTION _____ 10

What are Alzheimer's and Dementia? _____ 12

The Basics of the Mind Diet _____ 15

Planning Healthy Mind Diet Meals: 10 – Day Meal Plan _____ 20

Breakfast Recipes for the Mind Diet for Alzheimer's and Dementia _____ 21

Overnight Oats _____ 22

Whole Wheat Toast with Avocado _____ 23

Greek Yogurt Parfait _____ 24

Spinach and Feta Egg Scramble _____ 25

Chicken and Veggie Frittata _____ 26

Omelet with Mushrooms and Spinachs _____ 27

Blueberry Coconut Smoothie _____ 28

Steel Cut Oatmeal with Nuts and Berries _____ 29

Banana Walnut Pancakes _____ 30

Kale and Tomato Egg White Frittata _____ 31

Vegetable and Herb Frittata _____ 32

- Banana Oatmeal Bake _____ 33
- Tofu Scramble with Veggies _____ 34
- Apple Maple Walnut Oatmeal _____ 35
- Egg and Avocado Toast _____ 36
- Egg and Sweet Potato Hash _____ 37
- Chia Seed Pudding with Berries _____ 38
- Breakfast Parfait with Nuts and Seeds _____ 39
- Sweet Potato and Kale Breakfast Burrito _____ 40
- Quinoa Porridge with Berries _____ 41
- Breakfast Burrito with Black Beans and Rice _____ 42
- Kefir Smoothie with Berries _____ 43
- Granola with Yogurt and Berries _____ 44
- Egg and Kale Burrito _____ 45
- Lentil and Vegetable Frittata _____ 46
- Berry and Yogurt Smoothie Bowl _____ 47
- Egg White and Spinach Omelet _____ 48
- Baked Oatmeal with Apples and Walnuts _____ 49
- Chickpea and Spinach Scramble with Berries _____ 50

Lunch Recipes for the Mind Diet for Alzheimer's and Dementia _____ 51

- Quinoa and Black Bean Salad _____ 52
- Roasted Salmon with Spinach _____ 53
- Grilled Chicken Wrap with Hummus _____ 54
- Avocado and Chicken Salad _____ 55
- Bean and Veggie Burrito Bowl _____ 56
- Chickpea and Tuna Salad _____ 57
- Coconut-Lime Shrimp and Rice _____ 58

- Mediterranean Vegetable Frittata _____ 59
- Mediterranean Lentil Soup _____ 60
  - Broccoli and Cheese Stuffed Potatoes _____ 61
  - Mediterranean Baked Tofu _____ 62
- Turkey and Hummus Sandwich _____ 63
  - Egg and Avocado Toast _____ 64
  - Greek Salad with Chickpeas _____ 65
  - Roasted Vegetable and Feta Sandwich _____ 66
  - Quinoa and Roasted Vegetable Bowl _____ 67
- Shrimp and Veggie Stir Fry _____ 68
- Egg White Frittata with Spinach and Mushrooms _____ 69
  - Zucchini Noodles with Turkey Meatballs _____ 70
- Turkey and Spinach Roll-Ups _____ 71
- Veggie and Hummus Wrap _____ 72
  - Mediterranean Omelet _____ 73
  - Egg and Vegetable Salad _____ 74
- Hummus and Veggie Wrap _____ 75
- Salmon and Asparagus Quiche _____ 76
  - Greek Yogurt and Fruit Bowl _____ 77
- Lentil and Kale Soup _____ 78
  - Spinach and Feta Stuffed Chicken Breasts _____ 79
- Quinoa and Veggie Bowl _____ 80

Dinner Recipes for the Mind Diet for Alzheimer's and Dementia _____ 81

- Baked Salmon with Asparagus and Quinoa _____ 82
- Grilled Chicken Breast with Roasted Sweet Potatoes _____ 83
- Vegetable Soup with Lentils _____ 84

Cabbage and Bean Stew	85
Broiled Trout with Brown Rice	86
Grilled Veggie and Feta Cheese Wrap	87
Quinoa and Kale Salad	88
Baked Chicken with Roasted Vegetables	89
Spinach and Mushroom Omelet	90
Mediterranean Rice and Bean Bowl	91
Turkey and Spinach Stuffed Peppers	92
Steamed Fish and Vegetables	93
Roasted Vegetable and Farro Salad	94
Baked Halibut with Rice Pilaf	95
Roasted Tomato and Basil Soup	96
Greek-Style Chicken with Spinach	97
Grilled Haloumi Cheese with Zucchini	98
Chickpea and Spinach Curry	99
Mediterranean Chickpea Salad	100
Turkey and Black Bean Chili	101
Lentil and Veggie Stuffed Peppers	102
Baked Eggplant Parmesan	103
Broiled Halibut with Lemon and Tomatoes	104
Zucchini and Roasted Red Pepper Frittata	105
Grilled Vegetable and Quinoa Salad	106
Baked Salmon with Spinach	107
Shrimp and Vegetable Stir Fry	108
Roasted Vegetable and Feta Cheese Wrap	109
Baked Salmon with Lemon-Herb Sauce	110

Snack Recipes for the Mind Diet for Alzheimer's and Dementia ___ 111

- Avocado Toast with Sprouted Whole-Grain Bread ___ 112
- Roasted Chickpeas ___ 113
- Apple Slices with Almond Butter ___ 114
- Greek Yogurt with Berries ___ 115
- Trail Mix with Nuts and Dried Fruit ___ 116
- Roasted Veggies with Hummus ___ 117
- Kale Chips ___ 118
- Blueberry and Oat Smoothie ___ 119
- Dark Chocolate with Almonds ___ 120
- Edamame ___ 121
- Overnight Oats ___ 122
- Cottage Cheese with Fruit ___ 123
- Pumpkin Seeds ___ 124
- Cauliflower Tots ___ 124
- Fruit and Nut Bars ___ 126
- Hummus and Veggie Wraps ___ 127
- Popcorn with Olive Oil ___ 128
- Quinoa and Black Bean Salad ___ 129
- Celery Sticks with Peanut Butter ___ 130
- Salmon and Avocado Roll ___ 131
- Carrot Sticks with Tahini ___ 132
- Seaweed Snack ___ 133
- Coconut Yogurt with Granola ___ 134
- Banana Berry Smoothie ___ 136
- Apple Cinnamon Muffins ___ 137

Avocado Mousse	138
Baked Apple with Cinnamon and Honey	139
Blueberry Coconut Quinoa Pudding	140
Carrot Cake with Cream Cheese Frosting	141
Chocolate Chia Pudding	142
Coconut Yogurt Parfaits	143
Date Walnut Squares	144
Fruit Salad with Lemon Poppy Seed Dressing	145
Granola with Almonds and Raisins	146
Greek Yogurt Popsicles	147
Honeydew Melon with Mint	148
Lemon Poppy Seed Bars	149
Oatmeal Raisin Cookies	150
Peach Cobbler	151
Pear Crumble	152
Pineapple and Coconut Custard	153
Roasted Plums with Ricotta	154
Sliced Strawberries with Balsamic Glaze	155
Spiced Apple Cake	156
Strawberry Cream Cheese Pie	157
Trail Mix Bites	158
Vanilla Yogurt with Fresh Fruit	159
More Approaches to Managing Alzheimer's and Dementia	*160*
Conclusion	*162*

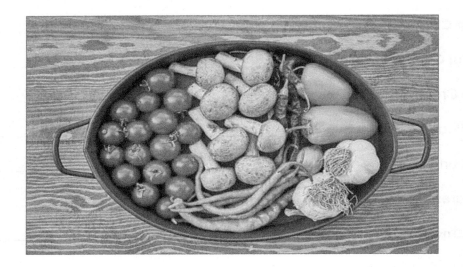

About the Writer

Zera Wright is the author of The Mind Diet Cookbook. She is a certified nutrition and fitness coach with a passion for helping people make positive changes to improve their overall health and well-being. She is also the founder and CEO of Nourish Yourself, a program that helps people learn how to make healthy, delicious meals that nourish their bodies and minds.

Zera believes that good nutrition is a key component of physical and mental health. She is dedicated to helping people make the right choices when it comes to their food and lifestyle. Through her cookbook, she offers readers delicious and easy-to-make recipes that are packed with nutrients, while also providing helpful information about the science of nutrition and how it affects the body.

The Mind Diet Cookbook provides readers with everything they need to make healthful and delicious meals, from advice on shopping and meal planning to step-by-step instructions for creating delicious dishes. With Zera's guidance, readers will be able to create meals packed with flavor and nutrition that will help them reach their health and wellness goals.

INTRODUCTION

Jesse had been overweight for most of his life and had been struggling with his health for years. He had high blood pressure and diabetes and was at risk of developing heart disease. After much deliberation, Jesse decided to undergo bariatric surgery to help him lose weight and improve his health.

The surgery was a success, and Jesse was able to lose a significant amount of weight. He was determined to keep it off and make the most of his new lease on life.

Phil was an active and vibrant 72-year-old retired banker who loved spending time with his family and friends. He was always up for a good game of golf or a round of cards. But one day, his life changed dramatically when he was diagnosed with dementia.

Phil's family was devastated. They wondered what they could do to help Phil and make his life better. After some research, they discovered the power of nutrition and the positive impact a healthy diet could have on neurological diseases like dementia and Alzheimer's.

This was the beginning of Phil's journey to find food that could fuel his brain and reduce the effects of dementia. He began to research the different diets available and eventually stumbled upon the MIND diet.

The MIND diet stands for Mediterranean-DASH Intervention for Neurodegenerative Delay, and it is a combination of Mediterranean and DASH diets. It focuses on specific nutrient-rich foods to reduce the risk of Alzheimer's and dementia.

This diet emphasizes the consumption of whole grains, leafy greens, nuts, berries, fish, and poultry. It also encourages the consumption of healthy fats, such as those found in olive oil, avocados, and nuts.

The MIND diet also recommends limiting processed foods, saturated fat, and sugar-sweetened beverages, as well as limiting red meat and full-fat dairy products.

It is important to remember that following this diet is not a guarantee that someone will not develop Alzheimer's or dementia. However, research has shown that following the MIND diet has been associated with a reduced risk of dementia and a slower rate of cognitive decline.

For Phil, the MIND diet was the perfect way to make sure he was getting the nutrients he needed to help him manage his dementia. He slowly began to incorporate the recommended foods into his diet and found that he felt much better. His family was amazed by the positive changes they witnessed in Phil and decided to create a cookbook to help others in similar situations.

Welcome to Mind Diet Cookbook for Alzheimer's and Dementia! This comprehensive cookbook is designed to provide you with nutrition information and meal ideas to help you feed your loved ones who struggle with Alzheimer's or dementia.

Alzheimer's and dementia are progressive diseases that can deeply affect the quality of life of a person living with them, as well as the lives of their family and friends. Nutritional health often takes a backseat when a person's cognitive abilities are declining, but it is an essential factor in managing the symptoms of these diseases. Eating a well-balanced diet rich in essential vitamins and minerals can aid in energy maintenance., as well as provide antioxidant protection and prevent malnutrition.

The Mind Diet Cookbook for Alzheimer's and Dementia provides dietary guidance and meal ideas for those living with dementia and Alzheimer's. It contains information about specific vitamins and minerals that may be beneficial for those living with these conditions, as well as recipes and ideas for meals that are easy to make and nutritious. It also includes information about foods to avoid or limit and tips for managing eating behaviors that can be common to those living with Alzheimer's or dementia.

The Mind Diet Cookbook for Alzheimer's and Dementia is a valuable resource for anyone wanting to ensure that their loved one living with Alzheimer's or dementia is receiving the best nutrition they can. We hope that this guide helps you to make informed decisions about what to feed your loved one and provides you with valuable information to help them stay healthy and nourished.

WHAT ARE ALZHEIMER'S AND DEMENTIA?

Alzheimer's

Alzheimer's disease is a progressive, degenerative neurological disease that affects millions of people around the world. It is characterized by memory loss, cognitive decline, and behavioral changes and is the most common cause of dementia. Alzheimer's Disease is a terminal condition with no known cure.

The exact cause of Alzheimer's disease is unknown., but it is believed to be caused by a combination of genetic and environmental factors. It is believed that some people may be more likely to develop the disease based on their genetic makeup. There is also some evidence that lifestyle factors, such as smoking and poor diet, may increase the risk of developing Alzheimer's Disease.

The symptoms of Alzheimer's Disease can be divided into three stages: early, middle, and late. During the early stage, patients may experience mild memory loss, difficulty concentrating, and confusion. As the disease progresses, symptoms such as disorientation become more severe, language difficulties, and changes in personality and behavior. During the late stage of Alzheimer's Disease, patients may experience severe memory loss, inability to take care of themselves, and difficulty communicating.

Diagnosis of Alzheimer's Disease is based on a combination of medical history, physical and neurological exams, laboratory tests, and imaging studies. A physician may order memory tests, such as the mini-mental state exam, to help diagnose the condition. In some cases, a lumbar puncture may be done to assess the presence of amyloid plaques, which are thought to contribute to the development of the disease.

Treatment for Alzheimer's Disease is aimed at managing symptoms and slowing the progression of the disease. Medications, such as cholinesterase inhibitors, can help improve memory, thinking, and behavior. Antidepressants and antipsychotics may also be prescribed to help manage symptoms. Non-drug treatments, such as occupational therapy and speech therapy, can help patients learn to cope with the changes brought on by the disease.

People with Alzheimer's Disease and their families face many challenges. There is no cure for the disease, and treatment is aimed at managing symptoms and slowing the progression of the disease. It is critical to remember that people with Alzheimer's disease can still live fulfilling lives., and there are many resources available to help them and their families. Support groups, counseling, and respite care are just some of the services available to help people cope with the condition.

Alzheimer's disease is a devastating condition affecting millions of people around the world. Although there is no known cure, there are treatments available that can help manage symptoms and slow the progression of the disease. People with Alzheimer's Disease can live a better life with the right support and resources.

Stages of Alzheimer's

Early-stage Alzheimer's is characterized by mild memory loss, difficulty in focusing and comprehension, and reduced problem-solving ability. In this stage, individuals may have difficulty performing tasks that require complex reasoning or multitasking and may also experience changes in their mood and behavior. At this stage, diagnosis is possible but not always definitive.

Middle-stage Alzheimer's is more severe and is characterized by increased memory loss and confusion, difficulty in communicating and understanding language, impaired judgment, and decreased problem-solving skills. In this stage, people may experience further changes in their mood and behavior, including increased agitation, restlessness, and paranoia. It is also possible for individuals to become socially isolated and dependent on others for their care.

Late-stage Alzheimer's is the most advanced stage of the disease and is characterized by significant memory loss, difficulty in recognizing familiar people and objects, and complete or near-complete dependence on others for basic daily needs. Communication abilities are severely impaired, and individuals may be unable to remember recent events or comprehend complex ideas. Many people in this stage also experience changes in their physical abilities, such as difficulty in walking or in carrying out basic tasks.

Dementia

Dementia is a degenerative neurological disorder that affects a person's memory, thinking, behavior, and ability to perform everyday activities. It is one of the most common neurological disorders among older adults, and the risk of developing dementia increases significantly with age. Dementia is not a single disease but rather a broad term used to describe a group of symptoms associated with a decline in cognitive function. Alzheimer's disease is the most common type of dementia, but there are others, such as vascular dementia, Lewy body dementia, and frontotemporal dementia.

The exact cause of dementia is not known, but there are several factors that may increase the risk. These include age, family history, lifestyle factors such as smoking and alcohol use, and certain medical conditions such as diabetes and high blood pressure. In addition, some medications and other environmental factors may contribute to the development of dementia.

The symptoms of dementia can vary depending on the type and severity, but they typically involve a decline in cognitive abilities, including memory, language, and problem-solving skills. Other common symptoms include difficulty with daily activities, changes in personality and behavior, and difficulty communicating. In some cases, the person may experience hallucinations or delusions.

The diagnosis of dementia is typically made by a doctor based on a thorough evaluation of the patient's medical and family history, as well as physical and neurological examinations. In some cases, additional tests, such as brain imaging, may be used to confirm the diagnosis.

Unfortunately, there is no cure for dementia. However, there are treatments available that can help manage the symptoms and slow the progression of the disease. These include medications to treat specific symptoms, therapies to improve communication and cognition, and lifestyle changes to help the person maintain an independent lifestyle. In addition, there are several support services available to help people cope with the disease and its effects.

THE BASICS OF THE MIND DIET

The Mind Diet is a dietary program that was developed to help promote optimal mental health and well-being. It is based on the Mediterranean style of eating, which is considered to be one of the healthiest diets in the world. The Mind Diet is a combo of the Dietary

Approaches to Stop Hypertension (DASH) diet, the Mediterranean diet, and the MIND diet, which stands for the Mediterranean-DASH Intervention for Neurodegenerative Delay.

The Mind Diet focuses on eating a variety of nutrient-rich foods that are known to promote optimal mental health. The diet emphasizes eating whole grains, fruits, vegetables, lean protein, and healthy fats. It also encourages limiting foods that are high in added sugars, trans fats, and refined carbohydrates.

The Mind Diet includes a variety of foods that are known to promote mental health and well-being. This includes dark leafy greens, berries, nuts, fatty fish, legumes, olive oil, and whole grains. These foods are rich in antioxidants, vitamins, minerals, and other nutrients that are important for brain health. Eating a variety of these foods can help to protect against age-related mental decline and reduce the risk of developing Alzheimer's disease.

The Mind Diet also encourages limiting foods that can potentially harm mental health. This includes processed and fried foods, red meat, and refined carbohydrates. These foods can increase inflammation in the body, which can lead to a variety of mental health issues. Eating a diet that is free of these foods can help to reduce inflammation and improve overall mental health.

Along with consuming a variety of nutritious foods, the Mind Diet also encourages making lifestyle changes that can promote mental health. This includes getting enough sleep, managing stress, staying active, and engaging in activities that promote positive mental health.

Overall, the Mind Diet is a great way to promote optimal mental health and well-being. It encourages eating a variety of nutrient-rich foods while limiting processed and unhealthy foods. In addition, it encourages making lifestyle changes that can also improve mental health. Following the Mind Diet can help to reduce the risk of age-related mental decline and improve overall mental health and well-being.

The Mind Diet is not a miracle cure for mental health issues, but it can be a great way to support optimal mental health. Eating a variety of nutrient-rich foods and making lifestyle changes can help to protect against age-related mental decline and reduce the risk of developing Alzheimer's disease. Following the Mind Diet can also help to improve overall mental health and well-being.

WHAT ARE THE BENEFITS OF THE MIND DIET?

The Mind Diet has several potential benefits for people who follow it, including:

1. Lower risk of Alzheimer's Disease and Dementia: The Mind Diet has been found to reduce the risk of developing Alzheimer's disease and other forms of dementia. In a study of over 900 participants, those who followed the Mind Diet had a 53% lower risk of developing Alzheimer's disease.

2. Improved Cognitive Function: The Mind Diet has also been found to improve cognitive function and delay cognitive decline. In a study of over 1,200 participants, those who followed the Mind Diet had significantly better scores on tests measuring cognitive function than those who did not follow the diet.

3. Improved Mood: The Mind Diet has also been found to improve mood. In a study of over 1,500 participants, those who followed the Mind Diet had significantly better scores on tests measuring mood than those who did not follow the diet.

4. Reduced Risk of Heart Disease: The Mind Diet has also been found to reduce the risk of heart disease. In a study of over 1,000 participants, those who followed the Mind Diet had a lower risk of developing heart disease than those who did not follow the diet.

TIPS FOR SUCCESSFULLY IMPLEMENTING THE MIND DIET FOR ALZHEIMER'S AND DEMENTIA

The Mind Diet for Alzheimer's and Dementia can be an effective way to reduce a person's risk of developing cognitive decline and dementia. This diet focuses on the intake of certain nutrient-rich foods and limiting the amount of unhealthy processed foods. To successfully implement the Mind Diet, it is important to take the time to create a plan and be consistent with it. Here are some tips to help ensure success:

1. Start slow: Making drastic changes to your diet can be overwhelming and difficult to stick to, so begin slowly by incorporating one or two healthy components of the Mind Diet at a time. For example, start by adding one serving of a leafy green vegetable or dark-colored fruit to your diet each day, and then gradually add more Mind Diet-friendly foods.

2. Find healthy substitutions: If you love a certain food that is not included in the Mind Diet, try to find a healthier alternative. For instance, if you are a fan of fried foods, you can use healthy cooking oil and bake the food instead.

3. Make it a lifestyle: To successfully implement the Mind Diet for Alzheimer's and Dementia, it is important to make the diet a part of your lifestyle and not just a short-term solution. Making small changes to your diet, such as cutting out processed foods and increasing the number of nutrient-rich foods, can help you stick to the diet in the long run.

4. Track your progress: Keeping track of your progress is a great way to stay motivated and help you make sure that you are getting the most out of the Mind Diet. Write down the foods you have eaten and any changes you have noticed in your overall health. This will help you stay on track and help you recognize areas where you may need to make further changes.

5. Talk to your doctor: For more personalized help and guidance, it is important to talk to your doctor about any questions or concerns you may have about the Mind Diet. Your doctor can help you design a healthy eating plan and provide additional resources to ensure that you are successfully implementing the diet.

The Mind Diet for Alzheimer's and Dementia is an effective way to help reduce a person's risk of developing cognitive decline and dementia. By taking the time to plan and be consistent with the diet, you can successfully implement the Mind Diet and make it a part of your lifestyle.

FOOD GROUPS OF THE MIND DIET

The MIND diet is a dietary pattern that is specifically designed to support brain health and reduce the risk of cognitive decline and dementia. It combines elements of the Mediterranean diet and the DASH diet and emphasizes the consumption of 10 key food groups. Here are the ten food groups of the MIND diet, along with explanations:

Green leafy vegetables: This group includes vegetables such as spinach, kale, collard greens, and broccoli. These vegetables are high in nutrients such as vitamin K, folate, and antioxidants, which have been linked to brain health.

Other vegetables: This group includes non-starchy vegetables such as carrots, tomatoes, peppers, and onions. These vegetables are also high in antioxidants and provide additional vitamins and minerals that support brain function.

Nuts: Nuts are a good source of healthy fats, protein, and fiber. They have been linked to lower rates of cognitive decline and are a good snack option for the MIND diet.

Berries: Berries are high in antioxidants and other nutrients that have been linked to brain health. This group includes berries such as blueberries, strawberries, raspberries, and blackberries.

Beans: Beans are a good source of fiber and protein and are a good alternative to animal-based protein sources. They have also been linked to lower rates of cognitive decline.

Whole grains: Whole wheat bread, brown rice, and quinoa are good sources of fiber and other nutrients that support brain health.

Fish: Omega-3 fatty acids, which are surplus in fish, have been associated with a slowed rate of cognitive decline. This group includes fatty fish such as salmon, tuna, and mackerel.

Poultry: Poultry such as chicken and turkey are a good source of protein and are lower in saturated fat than red meat. They are a good alternative to red meat for the MIND diet.

Olive oil: A healthy source of monounsaturated fat, which has been linked to brain health. It is a good alternative to other types of oils and fats.

Wine: Wine in moderation has been linked to lower rates of cognitive decline. This group includes red wine specifically, and it should be consumed in moderation as part of an overall healthy diet.

Overall, the MIND diet emphasizes the consumption of nutrient-dense whole foods that have been linked to brain health. It also emphasizes limiting the consumption of processed foods, saturated fat, and sugary foods and drinks. By following the MIND diet, you can support your brain health and reduce your risk of cognitive decline and dementia.

Planning Healthy Mind Diet Meals: 10 – Day Meal Plan

Day	Breakfast	Lunch	Snack	Dinner	Dessert
1	Greek yogurt parfait	Roasted vegetable salad	Sliced apple with almond	Grilled salmon with quinoa	Blueberry oat bars
2	Scrambled eggs	Tuna salad sandwich on whole-wheat bread	Baby carrots with hummus	Grilled chicken with sweet potato fries	Chocolate avocado pudding
3	Breakfast quinoa bowl	Greek salad	Edamame	Baked cod with mixed vegetables	Banana oat cookies
4	Green smoothie	Turkey wraps with avocado spread	Orange slices	Broiled salmon with roasted potatoes	Lemon sorbet
5	Omelet with vegetables	Minestrone soup with whole-grain bread	Greek yogurt with berries	Beef stir-fry with brown rice	Chocolate chia seed pudding
6	Overnight oats	Grilled chicken Caesar salad	Cherry tomatoes with mozzarella	Baked chicken with roasted vegetables	Apple crisp
7	Sweet potato toast	Lentil soup with whole-grain crackers	Sliced cucumber with tzatziki sauce	Grilled flank steak with roasted asparagus	Blueberry cobbler
8	Smoothie bowl	Turkey and cheese wrap	Almonds	Grilled shrimp with quinoa	Dark chocolate truffles
9	Veggie omelet	Chickpea and tomato salad	Sliced pear with cheese	Grilled pork chops with roasted Brussels sprouts	Lemon bars
10	Avocado toast	Roasted vegetable quinoa salad	Baby carrots with ranch dressing	Baked salmon with mixed vegetables	Berry crisp

Note: This meal plan is just an example and can be modified based on your dietary preferences and needs.

Breakfast Recipes for the Mind Diet for Alzheimer's and Dementia

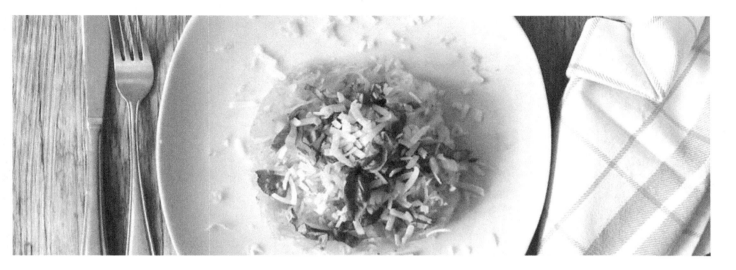

This section is full of delicious, nourishing breakfast recipes that are tailored specifically to the gastric sleeve bariatric diet. All of the recipes in this cookbook are rich in nutrients, low in calories and fat, and designed to help you stay full and satisfied throughout the day. Whether you're looking for a savory breakfast burrito, a protein-packed smoothie, or a light and fluffy omelet, you'll find something to love in this cookbook. So, let's get cooking and start the day off right!

Overnight Oats

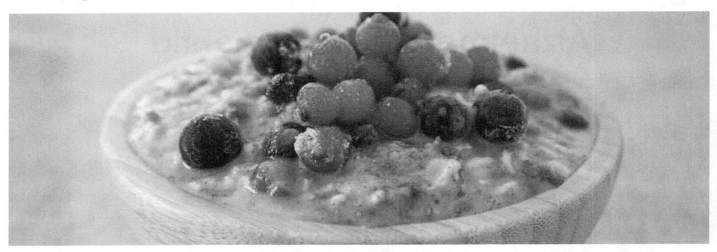

Ingredients

- ½ cup rolled oats
- ½ cup milk of your choice
- 1 tablespoon chia seeds
- 1 tablespoon honey
- 1 teaspoon vanilla extract
- Toppings of your choice (fresh fruit, nuts, nut butter, coconut flakes, etc.)

Instructions

- Combine oats, milk, chia seeds, honey, and vanilla extract in a bowl.
- Stir until combined.
- Cover and refrigerate overnight.
- In the morning, top with desired toppings and enjoy.

Whole Wheat Toast with Avocado

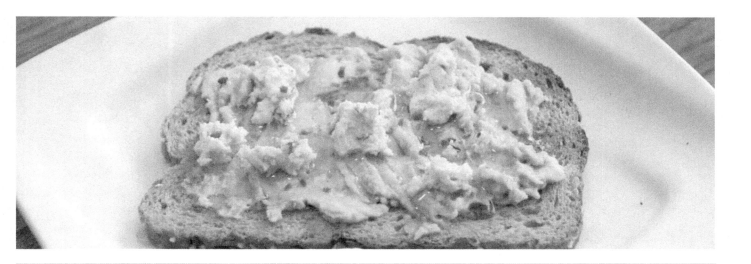

Ingredients

- 2 slices whole wheat bread
- 1 ripe avocado
- Salt and pepper to taste
- 1 tablespoon olive oil

Instructions

- Toast the bread until golden and crispy.
- Remove the avocado's pit and scoop out the flesh after cutting it in half.
- Mash the avocado in a bowl and season with salt and pepper.
- On the toasted bread, spread the mashed avocado.
- Drizzle with olive oil and enjoy.

Greek Yogurt Parfait

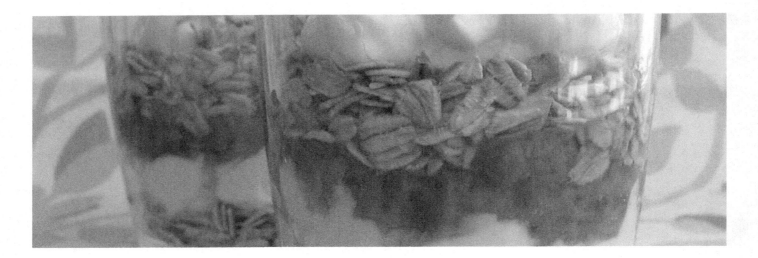

Ingredients

- 1 cup plain Greek yogurt
- 1 cup fresh fruit of your choice (berries, banana, kiwi, etc.)
- 2 tablespoons honey
- 1 teaspoon vanilla extract

Instructions

- Combine Greek yogurt, honey, and vanilla extract in a bowl.
- Stir until combined.
- Top with desired fresh fruit.
- Enjoy.

Spinach and Feta Egg Scramble

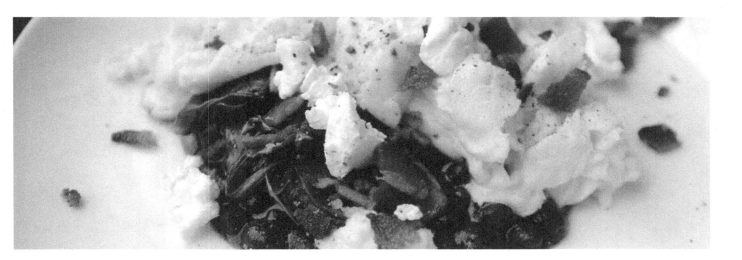

Ingredients

- 2 eggs
- 2 tablespoons milk
- ½ cup chopped spinach
- 2 tablespoons crumbled feta cheese
- 1 tablespoon olive oil

Instructions

- Heat the olive oil in the pan over medium heat.
- Beat eggs and milk in a bowl.
- Pour in the egg mixture and scramble until the eggs are cooked.
- Add spinach and feta cheese, stirring to combine.
- Cook until the spinach is wilted.
- Enjoy.

Chicken and Veggie Frittata

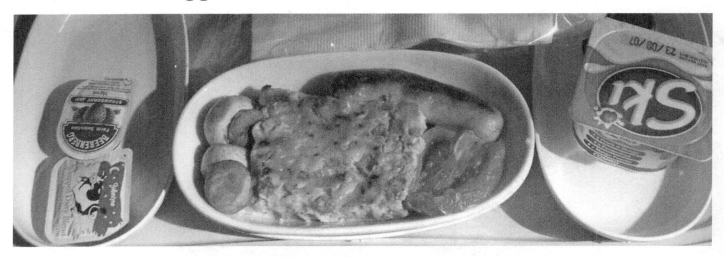

Ingredients

- 2 cups cooked and shredded chicken
- 1 red bell pepper, diced
- 1 cup frozen broccoli, thawed
- 1 cup shredded cheese
- 8 eggs, beaten
- Salt and pepper to taste

Instructions

- Preheat oven to 350 degrees F.
- Heat a 10-inch ovenproof skillet over medium heat.
- Add the chicken, bell pepper, and broccoli to the skillet and cook until the vegetables are tender.
- Add the cheese and stir until melted.
- Pour the egg mixture over the chicken and vegetables.
- Sprinkle with salt and pepper.
- Cook until the eggs are set, about 5 mins.
- In the oven, put the skillet, and bake for 10 minutes, or until the top is golden and the eggs are cooked through.
- Enjoy.

Omelet with Mushrooms and Spinachs

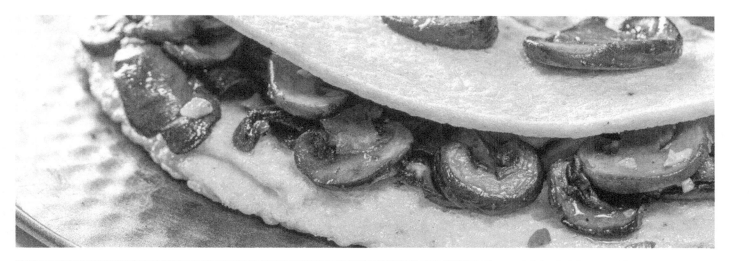

Ingredients

- 2 eggs
- 2 tablespoons milk
- 1 tablespoon butter
- ½ cup sliced mushrooms
- ½ cup chopped spinach
- ½ cup shredded cheese
- Salt and pepper to taste

Instructions

- Heat a nonstick skillet over medium heat.
- Beat eggs and milk in a bowl.
- Add the butter to the skillet and swirl to coat.
- Pour the egg mixture into the skillet and cook until the edges are set.
- Add the mushrooms and spinach, stirring to combine.
- Sprinkle with cheese.
- Cook until the eggs are set, and the cheese is melted.
- Fold the omelet in half and enjoy.

Blueberry Coconut Smoothie

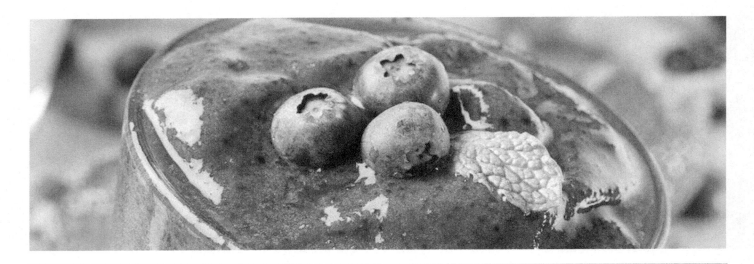

Ingredients

- 1 cup frozen blueberries
- ½ cup almond milk
- ½ cup coconut milk
- 2 tablespoons honey
- 1 teaspoon vanilla extract

Instructions

- In a blender, blend every ingredient until entirely smooth.
- Enjoy.

Steel Cut Oatmeal with Nuts and Berries

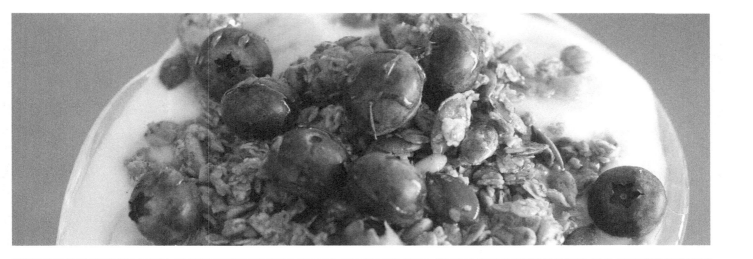

Ingredients

- ½ cup steel-cut oats
- 1 cup water
- ½ cup milk of your choice
- 1 teaspoon cinnamon
- 2 tablespoons chopped nuts of your choice
- ½ cup mixed berries
- 2 tablespoons honey

Instructions

- Combine oats, water, milk, and cinnamon in a saucepan.
- Boil the mixture, reduce heat, and simmer for 20 minutes, stirring occasionally.
- Add the nuts, berries, and honey.
- Cook for an additional 2 minutes.
- Enjoy.

Banana Walnut Pancakes

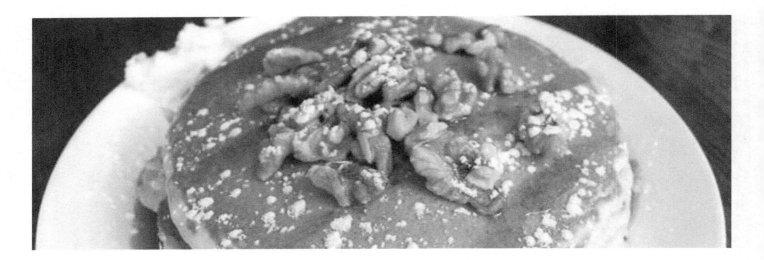

Ingredients

- 1 cup all-purpose flour
- 1 teaspoon baking powder
- ½ teaspoon baking soda
- ¼ teaspoon salt
- 1 ripe banana, mashed
- 2 tablespoons honey
- ¼ cup chopped walnuts
- 1 cup buttermilk
- 1 egg
- 2 tablespoons butter, melted

Instructions

- Mix the baking soda, flour, baking powder, and salt in a mixing bowl.
- Whisk together mashed banana, honey, walnuts, buttermilk, egg, and butter in a separate bowl.
- Pour the dry ingredients into the wet ingredients and mix until combined.
- Heat a nonstick skillet over medium heat.
- Grease the skillet with a bit of butter.
- Ladle ¼ cup of the batter into the skillet and cook until golden brown, flipping once.
- Repeat with the remaining batter.
- Enjoy.

Kale and Tomato Egg White Frittata

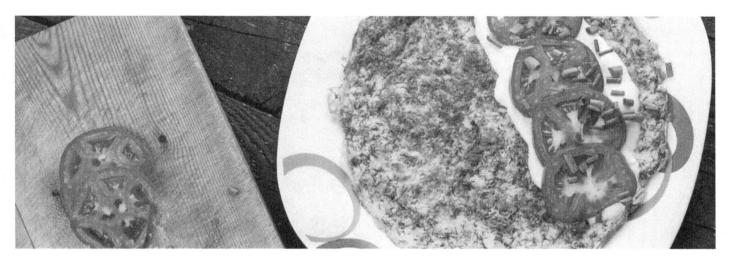

Ingredients

- 8 egg whites
- 1 cup chopped kale
- ½ cup diced tomatoes
- 2 tablespoons grated parmesan cheese
- Salt and pepper to taste

Instructions

- Preheat oven to 350 degrees F.
- Heat a 10-inch ovenproof skillet over medium heat.
- Beat the egg whites in a bowl.
- Add the kale, tomatoes, and parmesan cheese to the skillet.
- Pour the egg whites over the vegetables and stir to combine.
- Sprinkle with salt and pepper.
- Cook for 5 minutes, stirring occasionally.
- In the oven, put the skillet, and bake for 10 minutes, or until the top is golden and the eggs are cooked through.
- Enjoy

Vegetable and Herb Frittata

Cook Time: 25 minutes

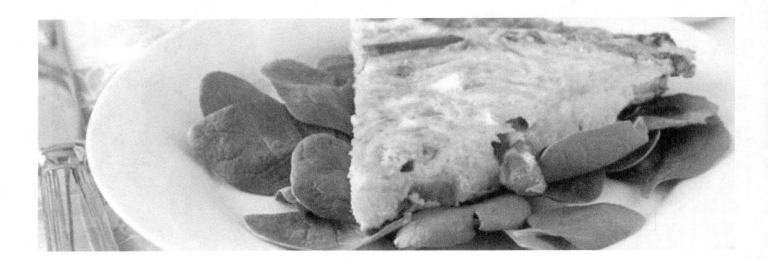

Ingredients

- 2 tablespoons olive oil
- 1 onion, diced
- 1 bell pepper, diced
- 1 cup of mushrooms, sliced
- 2 cloves of garlic, minced
- 4 cups of fresh spinach
- 2 tablespoons fresh herbs, such as oregano, basil, and thyme
- 8 eggs
- 1/4 cup of grated parmesan cheese
- Salt and pepper to taste

Instructions

1. Preheat oven to 350 degrees F.
2. Heat the oil in an oven-safe skillet over medium-high heat.
3. Add the onion, bell pepper, mushrooms, garlic, and spinach to the skillet and cook until the vegetables are softened about 5 minutes.
4. Add the herbs to the skillet and stir to combine.
5. In a bowl, whisk together the eggs, parmesan cheese, salt, and pepper.
6. Stir the egg mixture, then pour it into the skillet.
7. Place the skillet in the oven and bake for 15-20 minutes until the frittata is golden and set.
8. Serve warm.

Banana Oatmeal Bake

Cook Time: 45 minutes

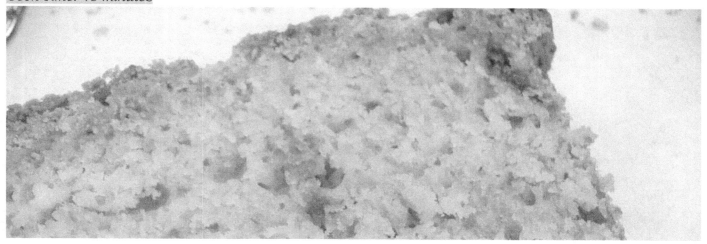

Ingredients

- 2 cups of rolled oats
- 2 ripe bananas, mashed
- 1/4 cup of chopped walnuts
- 1 teaspoon of ground cinnamon
- 1/4 teaspoon of salt
- 2 cups of milk
- 2 tablespoons of honey
- 2 tablespoons of melted butter

Instructions

1. Preheat oven to 350 degrees F.
2. In a bowl, combine the oats, mashed banana, walnuts, cinnamon, and salt.
3. In a separate bowl, whisk together the milk, honey, and melted butter.
4. Pour the dry ingredients into the wet ingredients and stir to combine.
5. Pour the oat mixture into a greased 8x8-inch baking dish.
6. Bake for 40-45 minutes until the oatmeal is golden and set.
7. Serve warm.

Tofu Scramble with Veggies

Cook Time: 45 minutes

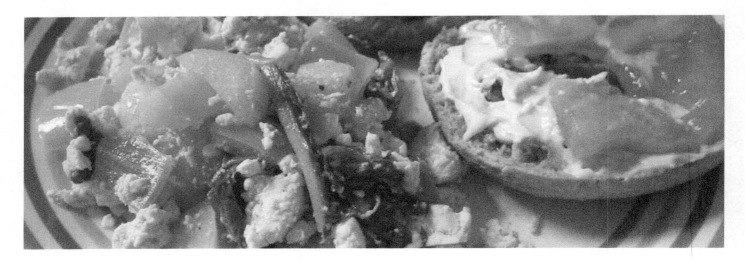

Ingredients

- 1 teaspoon of olive oil
- 1/2 onion, diced
- 1 bell pepper, diced
- 1/2 cup of mushrooms, diced
- 1/2 teaspoon of garlic powder
- 1/2 teaspoon of ground turmeric
- 1/2 teaspoon of ground cumin
- 1/4 teaspoon of salt
- 1/4 teaspoon of black pepper
- 1 block of firm tofu, crumbled
- 1/4 cup of shredded cheese (optional)

Instructions

1. Heat the oil in a skillet over medium heat.
2. Add the onion, bell pepper, and mushrooms to the skillet and cook until the vegetables are softened about 5 minutes.
3. Add the garlic powder, turmeric, cumin, salt, and pepper to the skillet and stir to combine.
4. Add the crumbled tofu to the skillet and stir to combine.
5. Cook for 5-7 minutes, stirring occasionally, until the tofu is heated through.
6. Remove from heat and stir in cheese, if desired.
7. Serve warm.

Apple Maple Walnut Oatmeal

Cook Time: 15 minutes

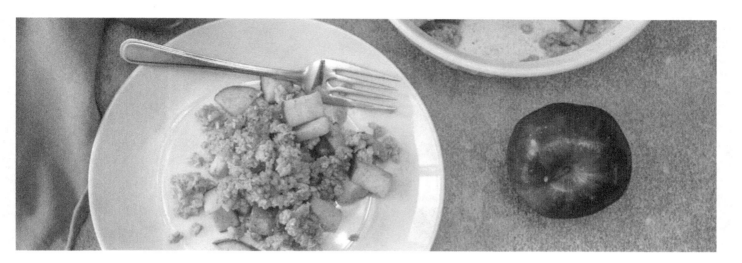

Ingredients

- 2 cups of rolled oats
- 2 cups of water
- 2 apples, peeled and diced
- 2 tablespoons of maple syrup
- 1/4 cup of chopped walnuts
- 1 teaspoon of ground cinnamon

Instructions

1. To begin, boil the water in a medium-sized pot.
2. Add the oats to the pot and reduce the heat to low.
3. Cook for 5-7 minutes, stirring occasionally, until the oats are cooked.
4. Remove from heat and stir in the apples, maple syrup, walnuts, and cinnamon.
5. Serve warm.

Egg and Avocado Toast

Cook Time: 10 minutes

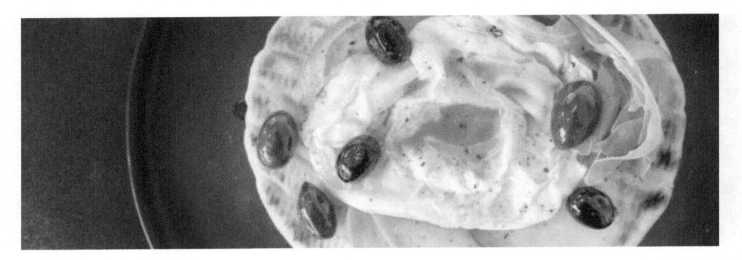

Ingredients

- 2 slices of whole grain bread
- 2 eggs
- 1 avocado, mashed
- 2 tablespoons of chopped cilantro
- Salt and pepper to taste

Instructions

1. Toast the bread in a toaster or in a skillet over medium heat.
2. Meanwhile, heat a non-stick skillet over medium heat.
3. Crack the eggs into the skillet and cook until the whites are set about 4-5 minutes.
4. Spread the mashed avocado onto the toast and top with the cooked eggs.
5. Sprinkle with cilantro, salt, and pepper.
6. Serve warm.

Egg and Sweet Potato Hash

Cook Time: 30 minutes

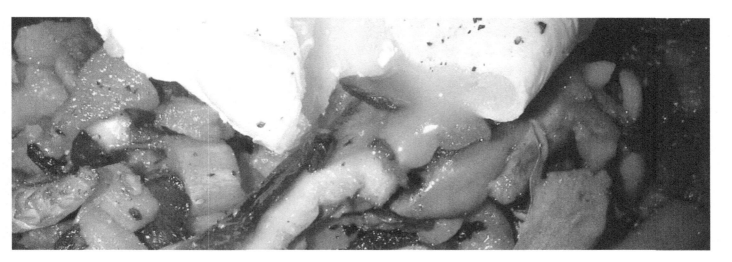

Ingredients

- 1 tablespoon of olive oil
- 1 onion, diced
- 1 sweet potato, peeled and diced
- 2 cloves of garlic, minced
- 2 teaspoons of smoked paprika
- 1/4 teaspoon of salt
- 1/4 teaspoon of black pepper
- 2 eggs

Instructions

1. Heat the oil in a skillet over medium heat.

2. Add the onion, sweet potato, garlic, paprika, salt, and pepper to the skillet and cook until the vegetables are softened about 10 minutes.

3. Make two wells in the mixture and crack an egg into each well.

4. Cover the skillet and cook until the eggs are cooked to your liking, about 5 minutes.

5. Serve warm.

Chia Seed Pudding with Berries

Cook Time: 15 minutes, plus 4 hours to chill

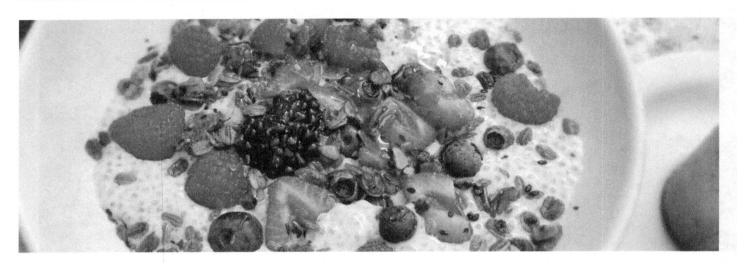

Ingredients

- 2 cups of almond milk
- 1/4 cup of chia seeds
- 2 tablespoons of honey
- 1 teaspoon of vanilla extract
- 1/2 cup of fresh or frozen berries

Instructions

1. In a bowl, whisk together the almond milk, chia seeds, honey, and vanilla extract.
2. Cover the bowl and refrigerate for at least 4 hours or overnight.
3. Divide the chia seed pudding into two bowls and top with berries.
4. Serve chilled.

Breakfast Parfait with Nuts and Seeds

Cook Time: 10 minutes

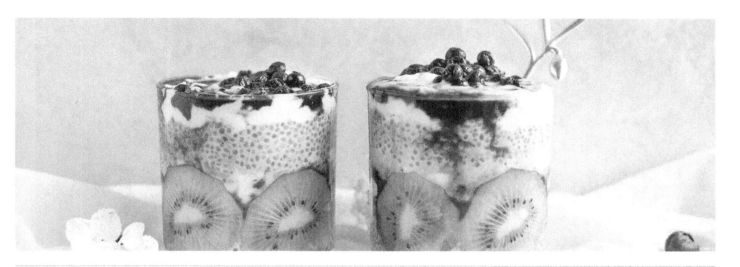

Ingredients

- 2 cups of plain yogurt
- 1/4 cup of chopped nuts, such as almonds or walnuts
- 2 tablespoons of chia seeds
- 2 tablespoons of hemp seeds
- 1/2 cup of fresh or frozen berries

Instructions

1. In two glasses, layer the yogurt, nuts, chia seeds, hemp seeds, and berries.
2. Serve chilled.

Sweet Potato and Kale Breakfast Burrito

Cook Time: 15 minutes

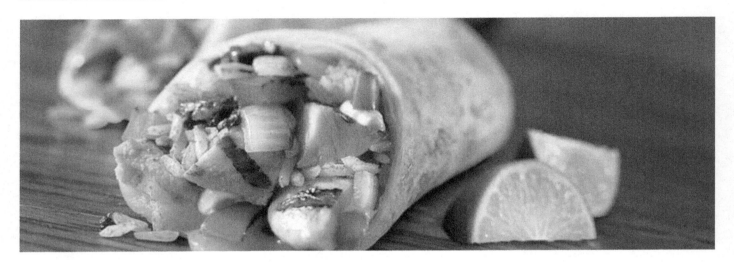

Ingredients

- 2 tablespoons of olive oil
- 1 sweet potato, peeled and diced
- 1/2 onion, diced
- 1/2 teaspoon of garlic powder
- 1/2 teaspoon of smoked paprika
- 1/4 teaspoon of salt
- 1/4 teaspoon of black pepper
- 2 cups of chopped kale
- 4 large eggs
- 4 large flour tortillas
- 1/2 cup of shredded cheese (optional)

Instructions

1. Heat the oil in a skillet over medium heat.
2. Add the sweet potato, onion, garlic powder, paprika, salt, and pepper to the skillet and cook until the vegetables are softened about 8 minutes.
3. Add the kale to the skillet and cook until wilted, about 3 minutes.
4. Crack the eggs into the skillet and stir to combine.
5. Cook until the eggs are cooked through, about 3 minutes.
6. Divide the mixture among the tortillas and top with cheese, if desired.
7. Roll up the tortillas and serve warm.

Quinoa Porridge with Berries

Cook Time: 20 minutes

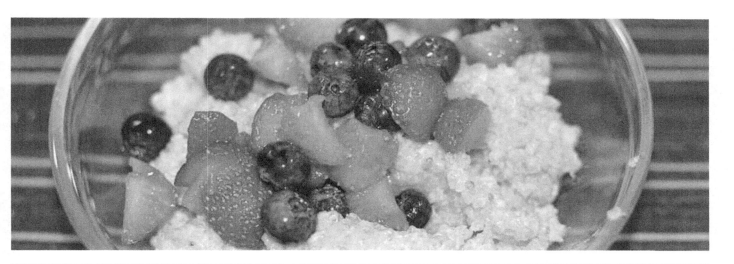

Ingredients

- 1 cup of quinoa, rinsed and drained
- 2 cups of water
- 2 tablespoons of honey
- 1 teaspoon of ground cinnamon
- 1/4 teaspoon of salt
- 1/2 cup of fresh or frozen berries

Instructions

1. Bring the water to a boil in a medium-sized pot.
2. Add the quinoa to the pot and reduce the heat to low.
3. Cook for 15-20 minutes, stirring occasionally, until the quinoa is cooked.
4. Remove from heat and stir in the honey, cinnamon, and salt.
5. Divide the quinoa among two bowls and top with berries.
6. Serve warm

Breakfast Burrito with Black Beans and Rice

Cook Time: 20 minutes

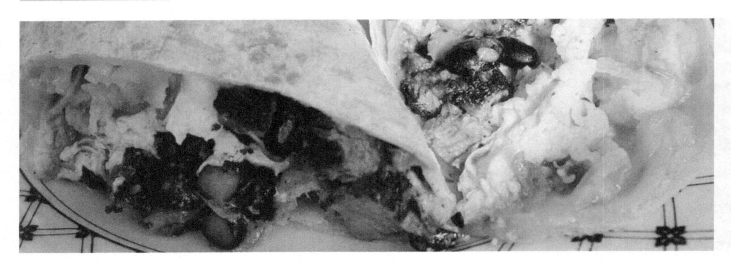

Ingredients

- 1 teaspoon olive oil
- 1 clove garlic, minced
- 1 cup cooked black beans
- 1 cup cooked white or brown rice
- 1/2 teaspoon ground cumin
- 1/4 teaspoon chili powder
- 1/4 teaspoon salt
- 1/4 teaspoon black pepper
- 4 large whole wheat tortillas
- 1 cup shredded cheese
- Salsa, for serving

Instructions

1. To begin, heat the olive oil in a medium skillet over medium heat.
2. Add the garlic and cook for 1 minute, stirring occasionally.
3. Add the beans, rice, cumin, chili powder, salt, and black pepper to the skillet and stir to combine.
4. Cook for 5 minutes, stirring occasionally.
5. Divide the bean and rice mixture among the four tortillas.
6. Top each burrito with 1/4 cup of shredded cheese.
7. Fold the sides of the tortillas in, then roll the burrito up.
8. Serve with salsa.

Kefir Smoothie with Berries

Cook Time: 5 minutes

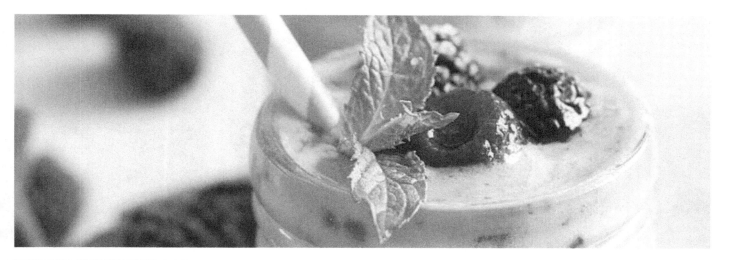

Ingredients

- 1 cup plain kefir
- 1/2 cup frozen mixed berries
- 1/2 banana, sliced
- 1 tablespoon honey

Instructions

1. Place the kefir, frozen berries, banana, and honey in a blender.
2. Blend until smooth.
3. Pour into a glass and enjoy.

Granola with Yogurt and Berries

Cook Time: 25 minutes

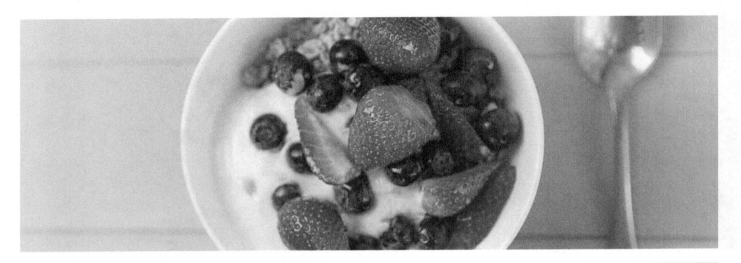

Ingredients

- 2 cups rolled oats
- 1/2 cup chopped nuts (almonds, walnuts, etc.)
- 1/4 cup shredded coconut
- 1/4 cup honey
- 1/4 cup coconut oil
- 1 teaspoon ground cinnamon
- 1/2 teaspoon ground nutmeg
- 1/4 teaspoon salt
- 1 cup plain Greek yogurt
- 1 cup fresh or frozen berries

Instructions

1. Preheat oven to 350°F.
2. Combine the oats, nuts, coconut, honey, coconut oil, cinnamon, nutmeg, and salt in a large bowl
3. Spread the mixture onto a baking sheet lined with parchment paper.
4. Bake for 20 minutes, stirring every 5 minutes.
5. Remove from oven and let cool for 5 minutes.
6. Place yogurt in a bowl and top with the granola and berries.
7. Enjoy!

Egg and Kale Burrito

Cook Time: 10 minutes

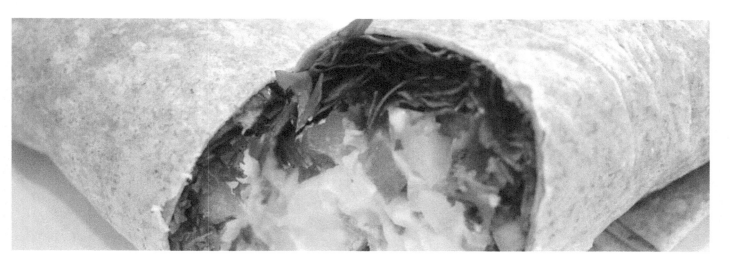

Ingredients

- 1 teaspoon olive oil
- 1/2 cup chopped onion
- 1/2 cup chopped bell pepper
- 1/2 cup chopped kale
- 3 eggs, beaten
- 1/4 teaspoon salt
- 1/4 teaspoon black pepper
- 4 large whole wheat tortillas
- 1/2 cup shredded cheese
- Salsa, for serving

Instructions

1. To begin, heat the olive oil in a medium skillet over medium heat.
2. Add the onion and bell pepper and cook until softened, about 3 minutes.
3. Add the kale and cook for 1 minute, stirring occasionally.
4. Pour in the eggs and season with salt and black pepper.
5. Cook until the eggs are set, about 5 minutes.
6. Divide the egg mixture among the four tortillas.
7. Top each burrito with 1/4 cup of shredded cheese.
8. Fold the sides of the tortillas in, then roll the burrito up.
9. Serve with salsa.

Lentil and Vegetable Frittata

Cook Time: 30 minutes

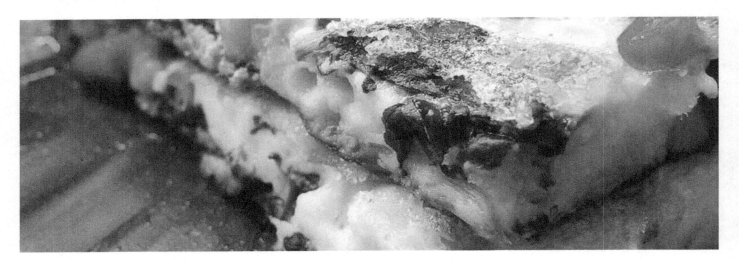

Ingredients

- 1 teaspoon olive oil
- 1/2 cup chopped onion
- 1/2 cup chopped bell pepper
- 1/2 cup cooked lentils
- 1/2 cup diced tomatoes
- 1/2 teaspoon dried oregano
- 1/2 teaspoon dried basil
- 6 eggs, beaten
- 1/4 teaspoon salt
- 1/4 teaspoon black pepper

Instructions

1. Preheat oven to 375°F.
2. Heat the olive oil in a medium skillet over medium heat.
3. Add the onion and bell pepper and cook until softened, about 3 minutes.
4. Add the lentils, tomatoes, oregano, and basil and cook for 1 minute, stirring occasionally.
5. Pour in the eggs and season with salt and black pepper.
6. Cook until the eggs are set, about 5 minutes.
7. Transfer the mixture to a baking dish.
8. Bake for 15 minutes or until the frittata is set.
9. Slice and serve.

Berry and Yogurt Smoothie Bowl

Cook Time: 5 minutes

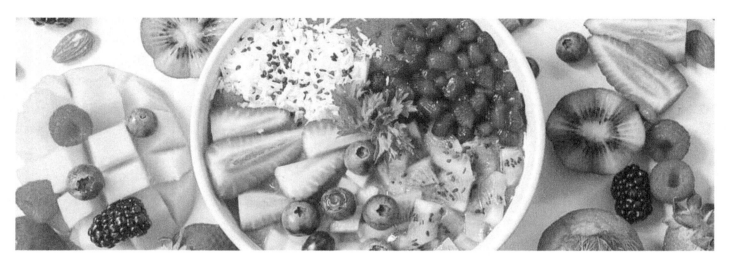

Ingredients

- 1 cup plain yogurt
- 1/2 cup frozen berries
- 1/2 banana, sliced
- 1 tablespoon honey
- 1/4 cup chopped nuts
- 1/4 cup shredded coconut

Instructions

1. Place the yogurt, frozen berries, banana, and honey in a blender.
2. Blend until smooth.
3. Pour the smoothie into a bowl.
4. Top with chopped nuts and shredded coconut.
5. Enjoy!

Egg White and Spinach Omelet

Cook Time: 10 minutes

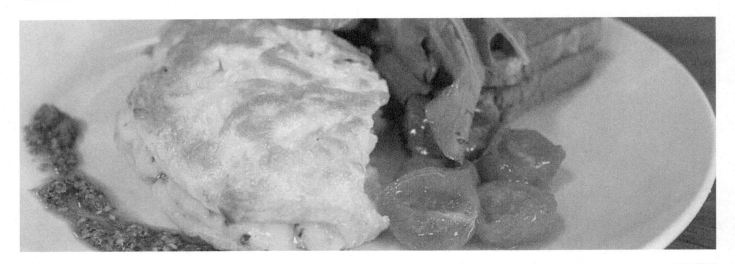

Ingredients

- 3 egg whites
- 1/4 cup chopped spinach
- 1/4 cup shredded cheese
- 1/4 teaspoon salt
- 1/4 teaspoon black pepper

Instructions

1. Heat a nonstick skillet over medium heat.
2. In a medium bowl, whisk the egg whites until frothy.
3. Add the spinach, cheese, salt, and black pepper and whisk to combine.
4. Proceed by pouring the egg mixture into the skillet and cook until the eggs are set, about 5 minutes.
5. Flip the omelet and cook for an additional 2 minutes.
6. Slice and serve.

Baked Oatmeal with Apples and Walnuts

Cook Time: 40 minutes

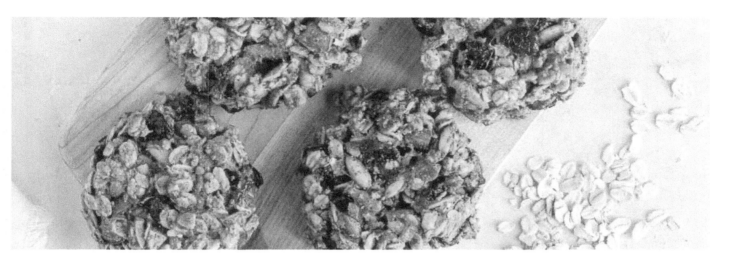

Ingredients

- 2 cups rolled oats
- 1/2 cup chopped walnuts
- 1/4 cup honey
- 1 teaspoon ground cinnamon
- 1/4 teaspoon ground nutmeg
- 1/4 teaspoon salt
- 2 cups apples, peeled and diced
- 1 1/2 cups milk

Instructions

1. Preheat oven to 350°F.
2. Combine the oats, walnuts, honey, cinnamon, nutmeg, and salt in a large bowl.
3. Stir in the apples and milk.
4. Transfer the mixture to a 9x13-inch baking dish.
5. Bake for 30 minutes or until the oatmeal is golden brown.
6. Enjoy!

Chickpea and Spinach Scramble with Berries

Cook Time: 10 minutes

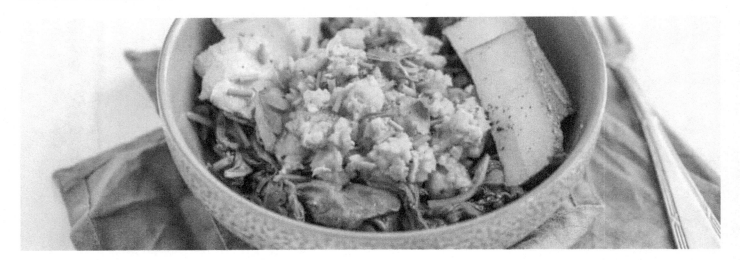

Ingredients

- 1 teaspoon olive oil
- 1/2 cup chopped onion
- 1 cup cooked chickpeas
- 1/2 cup chopped spinach
- 1/4 teaspoon salt
- 1/4 teaspoon black pepper
- 1/2 cup frozen berries

Instructions

1. To begin, heat the olive oil in a medium skillet over medium heat.
2. Add the onion and cook until softened, about 3 minutes.
3. Add the chickpeas, spinach, salt, and black pepper and cook for 2 minutes, stirring occasionally.
4. Add the frozen berries and cook for an additional 2 minutes.
5. Serve hot.!

Lunch Recipes for the Mind Diet for Alzheimer's and Dementia

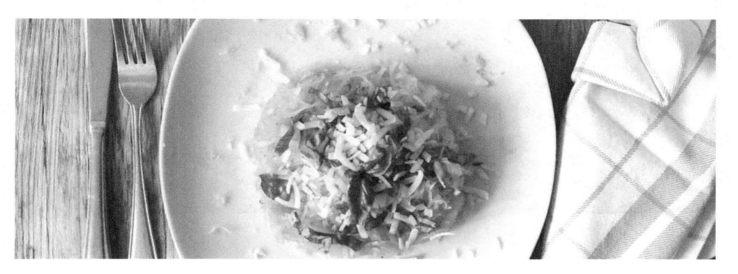

Lunch is an essential meal of the day that provides energy and nutrients to keep the body and brain functioning properly. For individuals with Alzheimer's and dementia, it is essential to include brain-healthy foods in their lunch recipes. The Mind Diet, which emphasizes on whole foods, has shown potential in reducing the risk of cognitive decline.

Quinoa and Black Bean Salad

Cook Time: 15-20 minutes

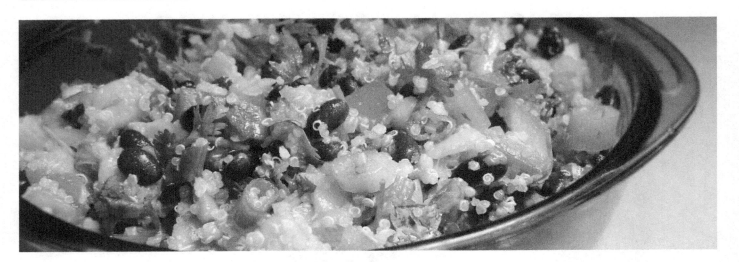

Ingredients

- 1 cup quinoa
- 1 can black beans, rinsed and drained
- 1 red bell pepper, diced
- 1/2 cup red onion, diced
- 2 cloves garlic, minced
- 2 tablespoons olive oil
- 2 tablespoons lime juice
- 1 teaspoon cumin
- 1/2 teaspoon chili powder
- Salt and pepper to taste

Instructions

1. In a medium pot, bring 2 cups of water to a boil. Add the quinoa, reduce heat to low, cover, and simmer for 15-20 minutes or until all the water is absorbed.

2. Combine the black beans, red bell pepper, red onion, garlic, olive oil, lime juice, cumin, chili powder, salt, and pepper in a large bowl.

3. When the quinoa is finished cooking, fluff it with a fork and add it to the bowl with the other ingredients.

4. Stir everything together until well combined. Serve warm or cold.

5. Enjoy!

Roasted Salmon with Spinach

Cook Time: 20 minutes

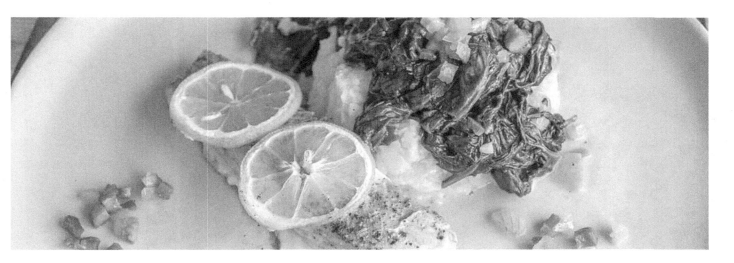

Ingredients

- 2 salmon fillets
- 2 tablespoons olive oil
- 2 cloves garlic, minced
- 1 teaspoon dried oregano
- 1/2 teaspoon dried thyme
- Salt and pepper to taste
- 2 cups baby spinach leaves

Instructions

1. Preheat oven to 400°F.
2. Onto a baking sheet lined with parchment paper. Place the salmon fillets
3. Drizzle the olive oil over the salmon and season with garlic, oregano, thyme, salt, and pepper.
4. Bake for 15-20 minutes or until the salmon is cooked through.
5. Meanwhile, place the spinach in a large bowl and set aside.
6. When the salmon is finished cooking, remove it from the oven and place it on top of the spinach.
7. Drizzle the remaining olive oil and juices from the baking sheet over the salmon and spinach.
8. Serve warm. Enjoy!

Grilled Chicken Wrap with Hummus

Cook Time: 15 minutes

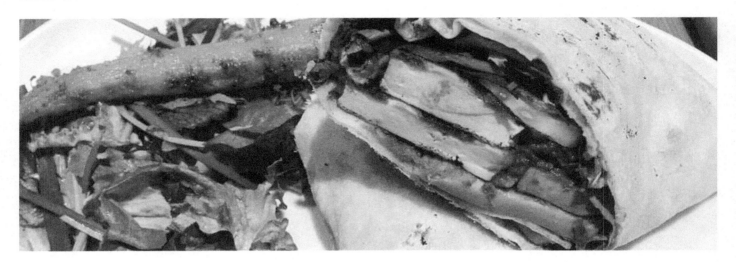

Ingredients

- 2 chicken breasts, pounded thin
- 2 tablespoons olive oil
- 1 teaspoon paprika
- 1/2 teaspoon garlic powder
- Salt and pepper to taste
- 2 wraps (flour or gluten-free)
- 2 tablespoons hummus
- 1/2 cup shredded carrots
- 1/2 cup shredded lettuce
- 1/4 cup feta cheese

Instructions

1. To begin, reheat a grill or grill pan to medium-high heat.

2. Brush the chicken breasts with olive oil and season with paprika, garlic powder, salt, and pepper.

3. Place the chicken on the grill and cook for 6-8 minutes per side or until cooked through.

4. Meanwhile, spread the hummus on the wraps.

5. Once the chicken is cooked, top the wraps with the chicken, carrots, lettuce, and feta cheese.

6. Roll the wraps up and enjoy!

Avocado and Chicken Salad

Cook Time: 15 minutes

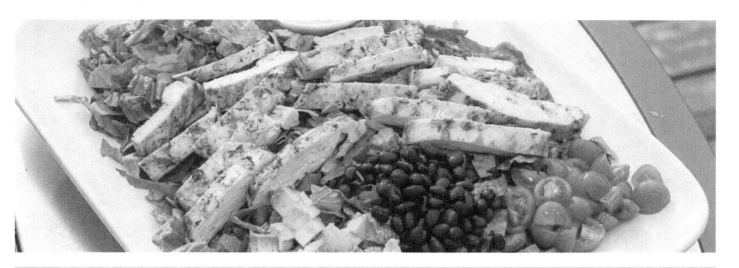

Ingredients

- 2 boneless, skinless chicken breasts
- 2 tablespoons olive oil
- Salt and pepper to taste
- 1 avocado, diced
- 1/2 cup cherry tomatoes, halved
- 1/4 cup red onion, diced
- 2 tablespoons lime juice
- 2 tablespoons cilantro, chopped

Instructions

1. Begin by preheating a grill or grill pan to medium-high heat.
2. Brush the chicken breasts with olive oil and season with salt and pepper.
3. On the grill, place the chicken and cook for 6-8 minutes per side or until cooked through.
4. Meanwhile, in a large bowl, combine the avocado, cherry tomatoes, red onion, lime juice, and cilantro.
5. Once the chicken is cooked, dice it and add it to the bowl.
6. Gently stir everything together.
7. Serve warm or cold. Enjoy!

Bean and Veggie Burrito Bowl

Cook Time: 20 minutes

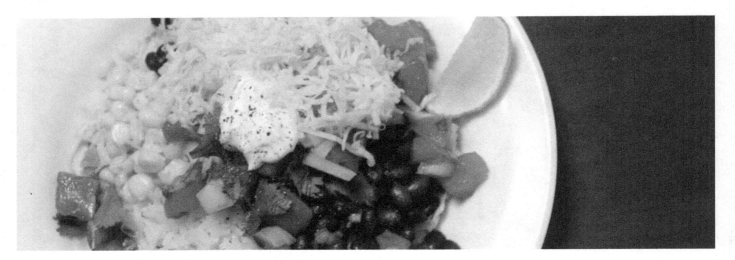

Ingredients

- 1/2 cup uncooked brown rice
- 1 can black beans, rinsed and drained
- 1 red bell pepper, diced
- 1/2 cup red onion, diced
- 1/4 cup frozen corn
- 1 tablespoon olive oil
- 2 cloves garlic, minced
- 1 teaspoon cumin
- 1/2 teaspoon chili powder
- Salt and pepper to taste

Instructions

1. In a medium pot, bring 1 cup of water to a boil. Add the brown rice, reduce heat to low, cover, and simmer for 20 minutes or until all the water is absorbed.

2. Combine the black beans, red bell pepper, red onion, corn, olive oil, garlic, cumin, chili powder, salt, and pepper in a large bowl

3. When the rice is finished cooking, fluff it with a fork and add it to the bowl with the other ingredients.

4. Stir everything together until well combined.

5. Serve warm or cold. Enjoy!

Chickpea and Tuna Salad

Cook Time: 10 minutes

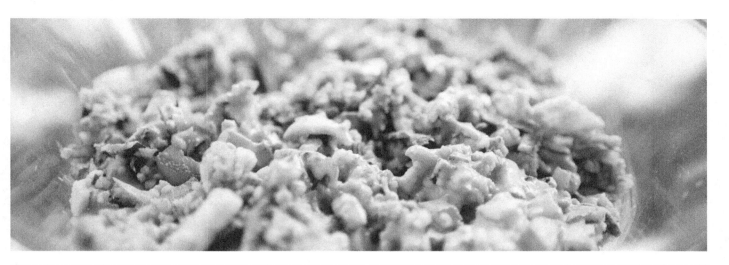

Ingredients

- 1 can chickpeas, rinsed and drained
- 1 can tuna, drained
- 1/2 cup red onion, diced
- 1/4 cup olive oil
- 2 tablespoons lemon juice
- 1 teaspoon dried oregano
- Salt and pepper to taste

Instructions

1. In a large bowl, combine the chickpeas, tuna, red onion, olive oil, lemon juice, oregano, salt, and pepper.
2. Gently stir everything together until well combined.
3. Serve cold. Enjoy!

Coconut-Lime Shrimp and Rice

Cook Time: 20 minutes

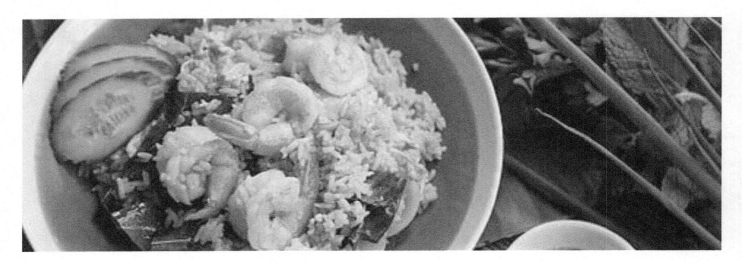

Ingredients

- 1/2 cup uncooked white rice
- 1 can of coconut milk
- 2 tablespoons lime juice
- 1 teaspoon curry powder
- 1/4 teaspoon cayenne pepper
- 1 tablespoon olive oil
- 1/2-pound shrimp, peeled and deveined
- 1/4 cup cilantro, chopped

Instructions

1. In a medium pot, bring the coconut milk, lime juice, curry powder, and cayenne pepper to a simmer.

2. Add the rice, reduce heat to low, cover, and simmer for 20 minutes or until all the liquid is absorbed.

3. Meanwhile, heat the olive oil in a large skillet over medium-high heat.

4. Add the shrimp and cook for 3-4 minutes per side or until cooked through.

5. Once the rice is finished cooking, fluff it with a fork and add it to the skillet with the shrimp.

6. Stir everything together and cook for 1-2 minutes.

7. Serve warm. Enjoy!

Mediterranean Vegetable Frittata

Cook Time: 25 minutes

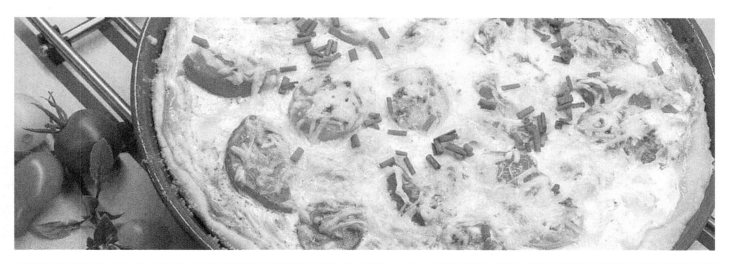

Ingredients

- 2 tablespoons olive oil
- 1 red bell pepper, diced
- 1/2 cup red onion, diced
- 2 cloves garlic, minced
- 2 cups baby spinach leaves
- 1 teaspoon dried oregano
- 6 large eggs
- 1/4 cup feta cheese
- Salt and pepper to taste

Instructions

1. Preheat oven to 350°F.
2. Proceed by heating the olive oil in a large oven-safe skillet over medium heat.
3. Add the red bell pepper, red onion, garlic, and spinach and cook until vegetables are softened about 5 minutes.
4. Add the oregano and season with salt and pepper.
5. In a large bowl, whisk together the eggs and feta cheese.
6. Pour the egg mixture into the skillet and cook for 5 minutes or until the edges are set.
7. In the preheated oven, place the skillet and bake for 15-20 minutes or until the frittata is cooked through.
8. Serve warm. Enjoy!

Mediterranean Lentil Soup

Cook Time: 30 minutes

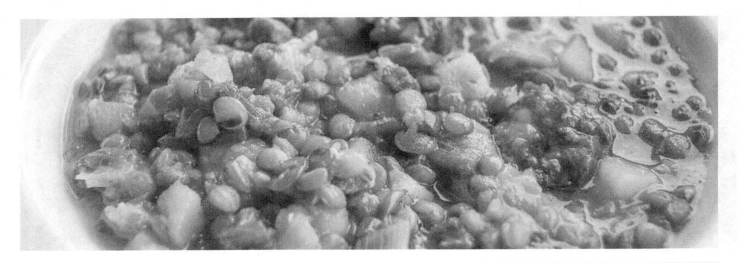

Ingredients

- 1 tablespoon olive oil
- 1/2 cup red onion, diced
- 2 cloves garlic, minced
- 1 teaspoon dried oregano
- 1 teaspoon dried basil
- 1/2 teaspoon dried thyme
- 1/4 teaspoon red pepper flakes
- 2 cups vegetable broth
- 1 can diced tomatoes
- 1 cup dry lentils
- 1/2 cup carrots, diced
- 1/2 cup celery, diced
- 2 tablespoons lemon juice
- Salt and pepper to taste

Instructions

1. To begin, heat the olive oil in a large pot over medium heat.
2. Add the red onion and garlic and cook until softened, about 5 minutes.
3. Add the oregano, basil, thyme, red pepper flakes, vegetable broth, tomatoes, lentils, carrots, and celery.
4. Bring the soup to a boil, reduce heat to low, cover, and simmer for 20 minutes or until the lentils are tender.
5. Stir in the lemon juice, salt, and pepper.
6. Serve warm. Enjoy!

Broccoli and Cheese Stuffed Potatoes

Cook Time: 30 minutes

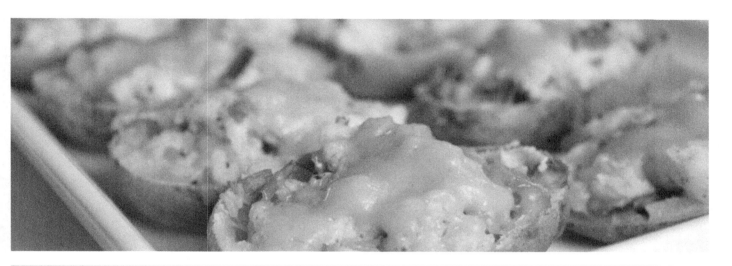

Ingredients

- 4 medium potatoes
- 2 tablespoons olive oil
- 2 cups broccoli florets
- 1/2 cup red onion, diced
- 2 cloves garlic, minced
- 1/2 cup shredded cheddar cheese
- 2 tablespoons butter
- Salt and pepper to taste

Instructions

1. Preheat oven to 400°F.
2. On a baking sheet lined with parchment paper. Place the potatoes
3. Drizzle the olive oil over the potatoes and season with salt and pepper.
4. Bake for 25-30 minutes or until the potatoes are tender.
5. Meanwhile, in a large skillet, heat the butter over medium heat.
6. Add the broccoli, red onion, and garlic and cook until softened, about 5 minutes.
7. Once the potatoes are finished cooking, cut them in half and scoop out some of the flesh.
8. Place the flesh in the skillet with the vegetables and mash together with a fork.
9. Stir in the cheese.
10. Stuff the potato skins with the mixture.
11. Serve warm. Enjoy!

Mediterranean Baked Tofu

Cook Time: 20 minutes

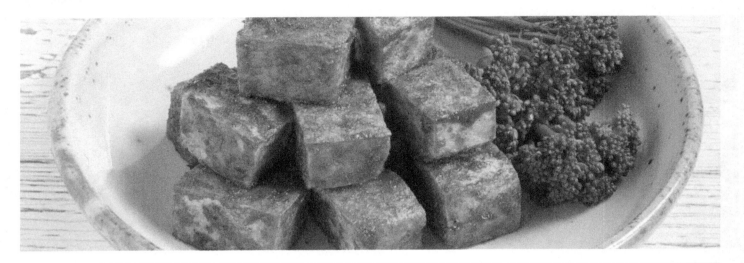

Ingredients

- 1 block extra firm tofu, cubed and drained
- 1/4 cup olive oil
- 1 tsp garlic powder
- 1 tsp oregano
- 1/4 tsp paprika
- 1/4 tsp black pepper
- 1/4 tsp red pepper flakes
- 1/4 cup sliced olives
- 2-3 tbsp capers

Instructions

1. Preheat oven to 375°F.

2. In a large bowl, combine the cubed tofu, olive oil, garlic powder, oregano, paprika, black pepper, and red pepper flakes. Mix until the tofu is evenly coated.

3. Spread the tofu onto a lined baking sheet and top with the sliced olives and capers.

4. Bake for 20 minutes.

Turkey and Hummus Sandwich

Cook Time: 10 minutes

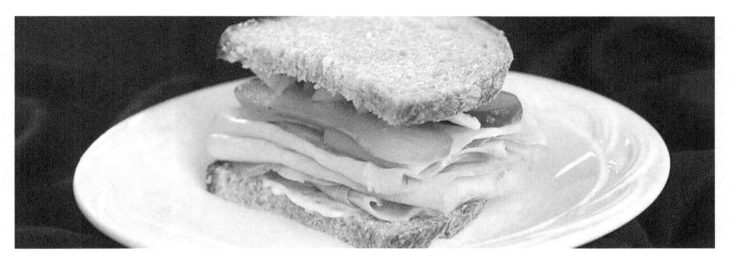

Ingredients

- 2 slices of whole wheat bread
- 2-3 tbsp hummus of your choice
- 2 slices of turkey
- 1/4 cup alfalfa sprouts
- 1/4 cup sliced red onion
- 1/4 cup sliced cucumber
- 1/4 cup sliced tomatoes
- Salt and pepper to taste

Instructions

1. Spread 1-2 tablespoons of hummus on each slice of bread.
2. Top one slice of bread with the turkey, alfalfa sprouts, red onion, cucumber, and tomatoes.
3. Sprinkle with salt and pepper to taste.
4. Top with the other slice of bread.
5. Cut in half and enjoy.

Egg and Avocado Toast

Cook Time: 8 minutes

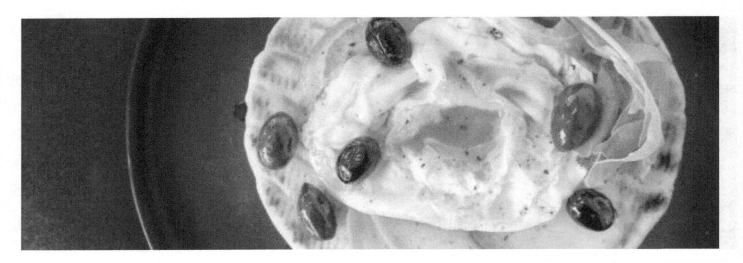

Ingredients

- 2 slices of whole wheat bread
- 1 avocado, mashed
- 1 tsp lemon juice
- 2 eggs
- Salt and pepper to taste
- 2 tbsp chopped fresh parsley (optional)

Instructions

1. Begin by toasting the bread to your desired level of crispiness.
2. In a bowl, mash the avocado and mix in the lemon juice.
3. Spread the mashed avocado on the toast.
4. Heat a skillet over medium heat and add the eggs. Cook until the desired doneness.
5. Place the eggs on top of the avocado toast.
6. Sprinkle with salt, pepper, and parsley (optional).

Greek Salad with Chickpeas

Cook Time: 15 minutes

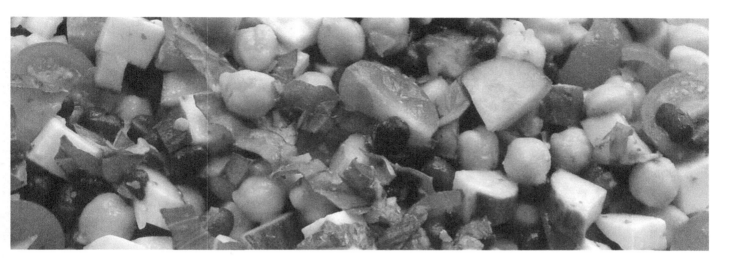

Ingredients

- 2 cups lettuce, washed and chopped
- 1/2 cup cherry tomatoes, halved
- 1/2 cup cucumber, diced
- 1/2 cup feta cheese, crumbled
- 1/2 cup black olives, sliced
- 1/2 cup cooked chickpeas, drained
- 2 tbsp olive oil
- 1 tsp red wine vinegar
- Salt and pepper to taste

Instructions

1. In a large bowl, combine the lettuce, tomatoes, cucumber, feta, olives, and chickpeas.

2. Whisk together the olive oil, red wine vinegar, salt, and pepper in a small bowl.

3. Proceed by pouring the dressing over the salad and toss to combine.

4. Serve and enjoy.

Roasted Vegetable and Feta Sandwich

Cook Time: 25 minutes

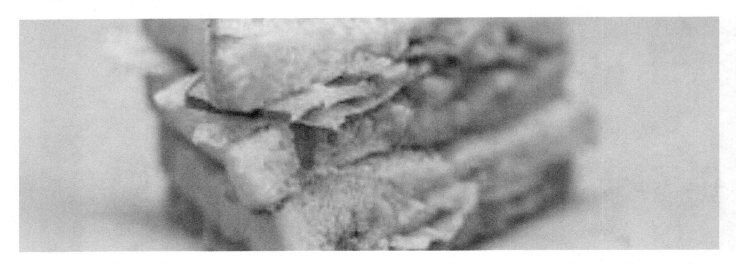

Ingredients

- 2 slices of whole wheat bread
- 1/2 cup roasted vegetables of your choice (ex: bell pepper, zucchini, eggplant, mushrooms, etc.)
- 2-3 tablespoons feta cheese
- 2 tablespoons pesto
- Salt and pepper to taste

Instructions

1. Preheat oven to 400°F.
2. Place the vegetables on a lined baking sheet and season with salt and pepper.
3. Roast for 20-25 minutes or until the vegetables are cooked through.
4. Spread one slice of bread with the pesto.
5. Top with roasted vegetables and feta cheese.
6. Sprinkle with salt and pepper.
7. Top with the other slice of bread and cut in half.
8. Enjoy.

Quinoa and Roasted Vegetable Bowl

Cook Time: 30 minutes

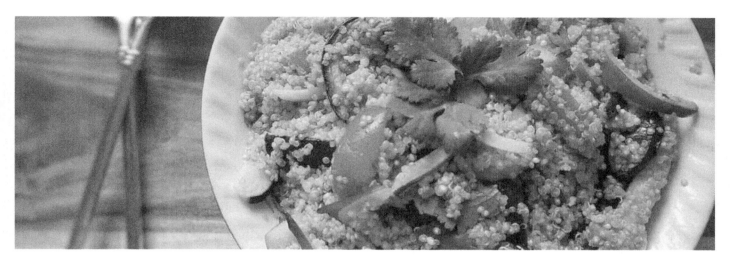

Ingredients

- 1 cup quinoa, cooked
- 1 cup roasted vegetables of your choice (ex: bell pepper, zucchini, eggplant, mushrooms, etc.)
- 1/4 cup crumbled feta cheese
- 2 tablespoons olive oil
- 1 tablespoon red wine vinegar
- Salt and pepper to taste

Instructions

1. Preheat oven to 400°F.
2. Place the vegetables on a lined baking sheet and season with salt and pepper.
3. Roast for 20-25 minutes or until the vegetables are cooked through.
4. In a large bowl, combine the cooked quinoa, roasted vegetables, feta, olive oil, red wine vinegar, salt, and pepper.
5. Mix until everything is evenly combined.
6. Serve and enjoy.

Shrimp and Veggie Stir Fry

Cook Time: 20 minutes

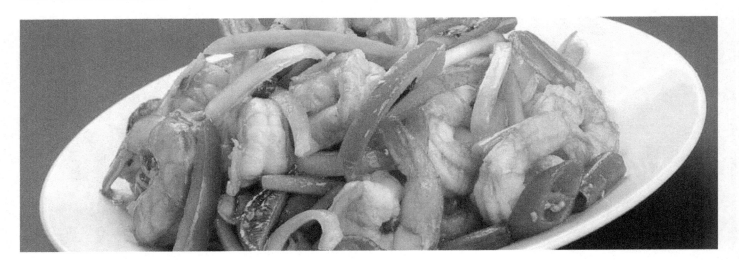

Ingredients

- 1 lb. shrimp, peeled and deveined
- 1/4 cup olive oil
- 1 onion, chopped
- 1 bell pepper, chopped
- 1 cup mushrooms, sliced
- 1 cup broccoli florets
- 2 cloves garlic, minced
- 2 tablespoons soy sauce
- 2 tablespoons sesame oil
- Salt and pepper to taste

Instructions

1. To start, heat the olive oil in a large skillet over medium heat.
2. Add the onion, bell pepper, mushrooms, broccoli, and garlic. Cook for 3-4 minutes.
3. Add the shrimp and cook for 3-4 minutes, or until the shrimp is cooked through.
4. Add the soy sauce and sesame oil.
5. Stir to combine and cook for an additional 1-2 minutes.
6. Season with salt and pepper to taste.
7. Serve and enjoy.

Egg White Frittata with Spinach and Mushrooms

Cook Time: 25 minutes

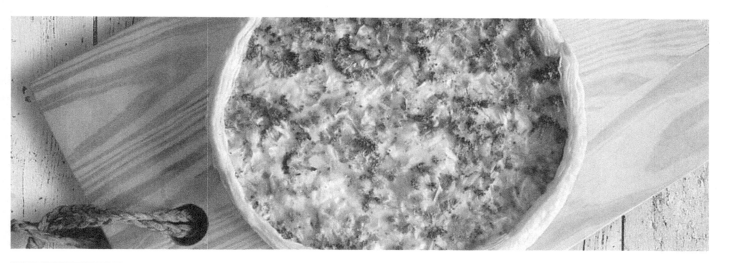

Ingredients

- 6 egg whites
- 1/4 cup skim milk
- 1/4 cup shredded cheese of your choice
- 1 cup spinach, chopped
- 1/2 cup mushrooms, sliced
- 1/4 cup red bell pepper, diced
- 2 cloves garlic, minced
- Salt and pepper to taste

Instructions

1. Preheat oven to 375°F.
2. Whisk together the egg whites and milk until combined in a large bowl.
3. Stir in the cheese, spinach, mushrooms, bell pepper, garlic, salt, and pepper.
4. Pour the mixture into a greased 9-inch pie plate.
5. Bake for 20-25 minutes, or until the frittata is set.
6. Serve and enjoy.

Zucchini Noodles with Turkey Meatballs

Cook Time: 25 minutes

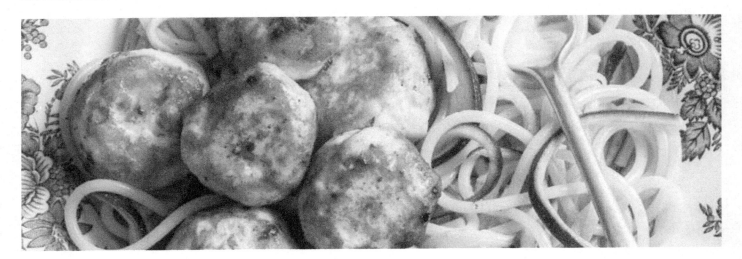

Ingredients

- 2 zucchinis, spiralized
- 1/2 lb. ground turkey
- 1/4 cup breadcrumbs
- 1 egg
- 1/4 cup grated Parmesan cheese
- 2 cloves garlic, minced
- 1 tsp Italian seasoning
- Salt and pepper to taste
- 2 tablespoons olive oil
- 1/2 cup marinara sauce

Instructions

1. Preheat oven to 375°F.
2. In a large bowl, combine the ground turkey, breadcrumbs, egg, Parmesan cheese, garlic, Italian seasoning, salt, and pepper. Mix until everything is evenly combined.
3. Form the mixture into small meatballs and place on a lined baking sheet.
4. Bake for 20-25 minutes, or until the meatballs are cooked through.
5. Heat a large skillet over medium heat and add the olive oil.
6. Add the zucchini noodles and cook for 2-3 minutes.
7. Add the marinara sauce and stir to combine.
8. Add the cooked meatballs and cook for an additional 2-3 minutes.
9. Serve and enjoy.

Turkey and Spinach Roll-Ups

Cook Time: 10 minutes

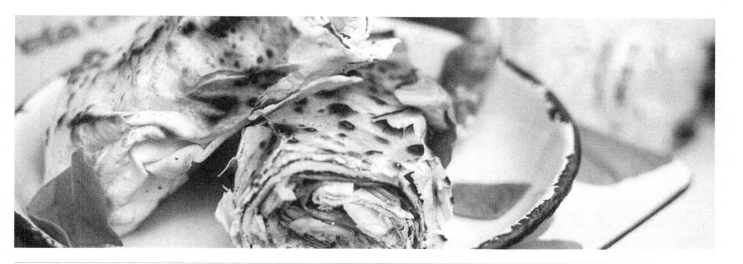

Ingredients

- 4 slices of whole wheat bread
- 4 slices of turkey
- 1/2 cup spinach leaves
- 2 tablespoons cream cheese
- 2 tablespoons shredded cheese of your choice
- Salt and pepper to taste

Instructions

1. Lay the slices of bread on a cutting board and spread each slice with cream cheese.
2. Top each slice of bread with spinach, turkey, and shredded cheese.
3. Sprinkle with salt and pepper to taste.
4. Roll up each slice of bread and cut it in half.
5. Serve and enjoy.

Veggie and Hummus Wrap

Cook Time: 10 minutes

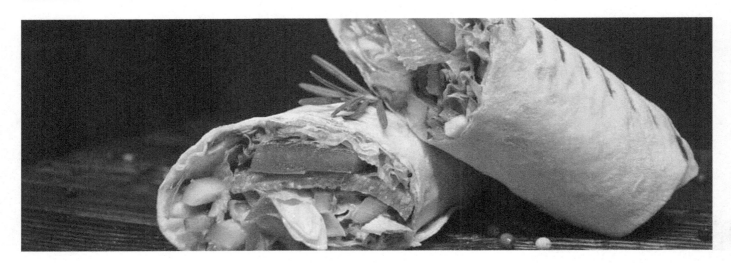

Ingredients

- 1 large whole wheat wrap
- ¼ cup hummus
- ¼ cup diced tomatoes
- ¼ cup diced cucumbers
- ¼ cup diced bell peppers
- ¼ cup cooked corn

Instructions

1. Place the wrap on a clean, flat surface.
2. Spread a thin layer of hummus on the wrap.
3. Top with diced tomatoes, cucumbers, bell peppers, and cooked corn.
4. Roll the wrap up tightly and cut it in half.

Mediterranean Omelet

Cook Time: 10 minutes

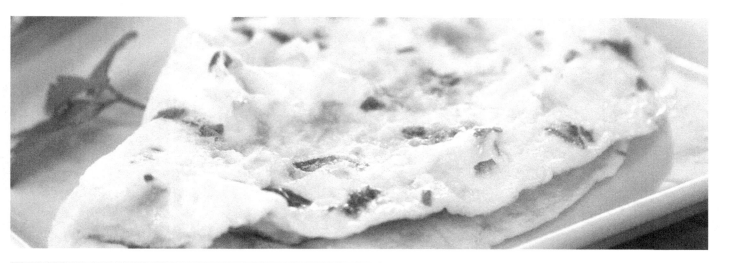

Ingredients

- 2 eggs
- 2 tablespoons milk
- 2 tablespoons diced bell peppers
- 2 tablespoons diced red onions
- 2 tablespoons diced tomatoes
- 1 tablespoon feta cheese

Instructions

1. Begin by whisking together eggs and milk in a bowl.

2. Heat a non-stick skillet over medium-high heat and spray with cooking spray.

3. Pour the egg mixture into the skillet.

4. Sprinkle bell peppers, red onions, and tomatoes over the top of the omelet.

5. Once the eggs are cooked through, sprinkle feta cheese over the top.

6. Carefully fold the omelet in half and cook for an additional 2 minutes.

7. Slide the omelet onto a plate and enjoy.

Egg and Vegetable Salad

Cook Time: 15 minutes

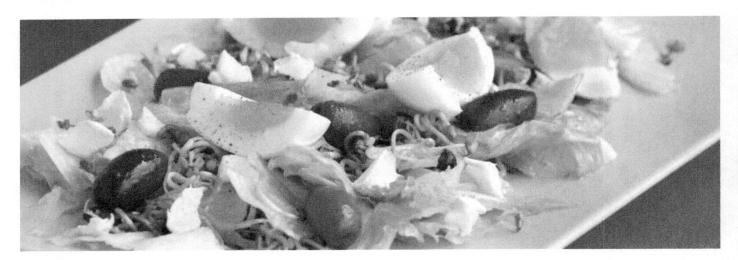

Ingredients

- 4 hard-boiled eggs, peeled and chopped
- 1 cup diced tomatoes
- 1 cup diced cucumbers
- ½ cup diced bell peppers
- ½ cup diced red onions
- ¼ cup Italian dressing

Instructions

1. In a large bowl, combine eggs, tomatoes, cucumbers, bell peppers, and red onions.

2. Pour Italian dressing over the top and stir until everything is evenly coated.

3. Refrigerate for at least 15 minutes before serving.

Hummus and Veggie Wrap

Cook Time: 10 minutes

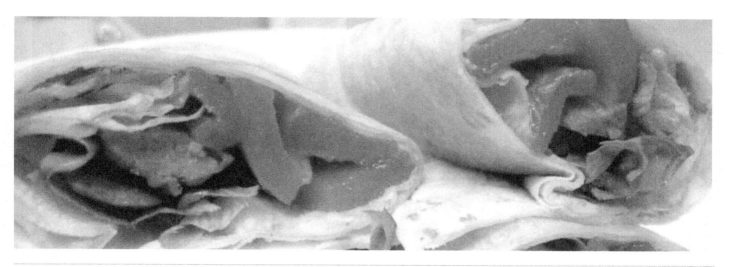

Ingredients

- 1 large whole wheat wrap
- ¼ cup hummus
- ¼ cup diced tomatoes
- ¼ cup diced cucumbers
- ¼ cup diced bell peppers
- ¼ cup cooked corn

Instructions

1. Place the wrap on a clean, flat surface.
2. Spread a thin layer of hummus on the wrap.
3. Top with diced tomatoes, cucumbers, bell peppers, and cooked corn.
4. Roll the wrap up tightly and cut it in half.

Salmon and Asparagus Quiche

Cook Time: 30 minutes

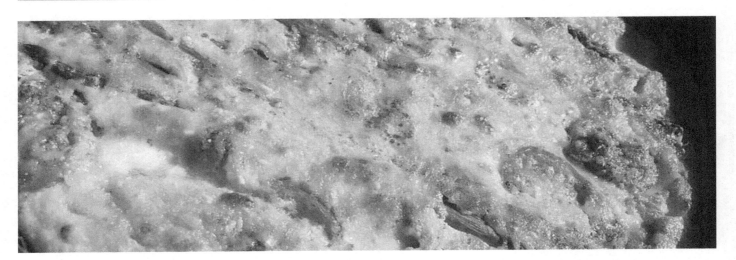

Ingredients

- 1 prepared 9-inch pie crust
- 1 tablespoon olive oil
- 2 cups cooked, flaked salmon
- 1 cup chopped asparagus
- 1 cup shredded cheese
- 4 eggs
- ½ cup milk
- Salt and pepper to taste

Instructions

1. Preheat oven to 375°F.
2. Heat olive oil in a skillet over medium-high heat.
3. Add salmon and asparagus to the skillet and cook for 5 minutes.
4. Place fish and vegetables in the prepared pie crust.
5. Sprinkle cheese over the top.
6. In a medium bowl, whisk together eggs and milk.
7. Pour the egg mixture over the top of the quiche.
8. Sprinkle with salt and pepper to taste.
9. Bake in the preheated oven for 25-30 minutes until the quiche is golden brown.

Greek Yogurt and Fruit Bowl

Cook Time: 5 minutes

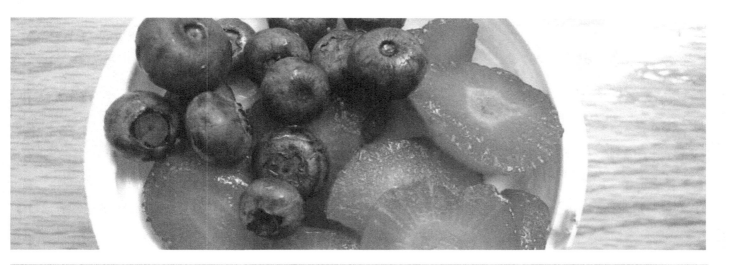

Ingredients

- 1 cup Greek yogurt
- 1 cup fresh or frozen fruit of your choice
- 1 tablespoon honey
- 1 tablespoon chopped nuts or seeds

Instructions

1. Place the Greek yogurt in a bowl.
2. Top with fresh or frozen fruit.
3. Drizzle with honey.
4. Sprinkle with chopped nuts or seeds.
5. Enjoy!

Lentil and Kale Soup

Cook Time: 45 minutes

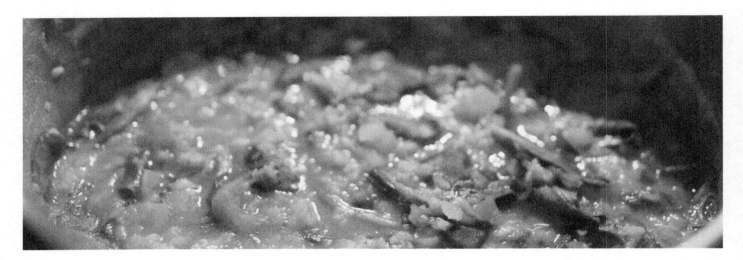

Ingredients

- 1 tablespoon olive oil
- 1 onion, diced
- 2 cloves garlic, minced
- 1 teaspoon dried oregano
- 1 teaspoon dried basil
- ½ teaspoon smoked paprika
- 2 cups vegetable broth
- 1 cup dry lentils
- 2 cups chopped kale
- Salt and pepper to taste

Instructions

1. Start by heating the olive oil in a large pot over medium-high heat.
2. Add the onion and garlic and cook until softened, about 5 minutes.
3. Add the oregano, basil, and smoked paprika and cook for an additional 1 minute.
4. Add the vegetable broth and lentils and bring to a boil.
5. Reduce heat and simmer, covered, for 30 minutes.
6. Add the kale and simmer for an additional 10 minutes.
7. Season with salt and pepper to taste.

Spinach and Feta Stuffed Chicken Breasts

Cook Time: 45 minutes

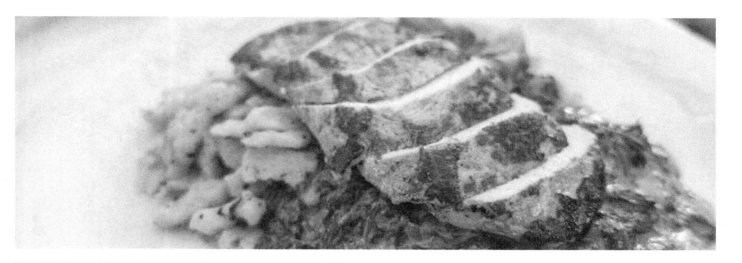

Ingredients

- 4 boneless, skinless chicken breasts
- 2 cups spinach, chopped
- ¼ cup feta cheese
- 2 tablespoons olive oil
- Salt and pepper to taste

Instructions

1. Preheat oven to 375°F.
2. Place chicken breasts in a baking dish.
3. In a medium bowl, combine spinach and feta cheese.
4. Divide the mixture among the chicken breasts, stuffing the mixture inside.
5. Drizzle chicken with olive oil and season with salt and pepper.
6. Bake for 40-45 minutes or until the chicken is cooked through

Quinoa and Veggie Bowl

Cook Time: 30 minutes

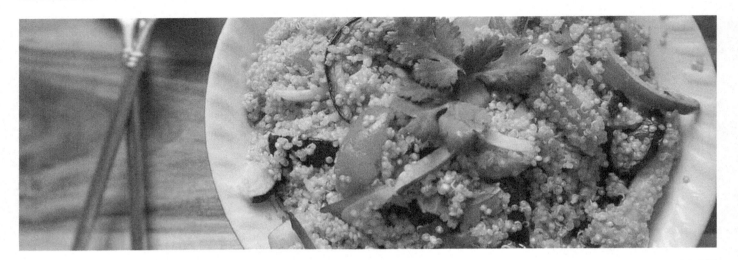

Ingredients

- 1 cup quinoa
- 2 cups vegetable broth
- 2 tablespoons olive oil
- 1 cup diced bell peppers
- 1 cup diced zucchini
- 1 cup diced yellow squash
- 1 cup diced mushrooms
- Salt and pepper to taste

Instructions

1. In a medium saucepan, combine quinoa and vegetable broth.
2. Bring to a boil, then reduce heat and simmer, covered, for 20 minutes.
3. Proceed by heating the olive oil in a large skillet over medium-high heat.
4. Add bell peppers, zucchini, yellow squash, and mushrooms and cook until vegetables are tender about 10 minutes.
5. Season with salt and pepper to taste.
6. To assemble the bowls, divide the quinoa and vegetables among four bowls.

Dinner Recipes for the Mind Diet for Alzheimer's and Dementia

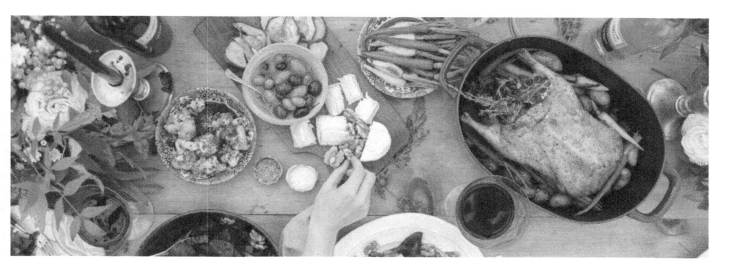

The Mind Diet is a dietary pattern designed to promote brain health and reduce the risk of cognitive decline, Alzheimer's, and dementia. Dinner is an essential meal of the day, and it plays a vital role in providing the body with essential nutrients and energy.

Baked Salmon with Asparagus and Quinoa

Cook Time: 30 minutes

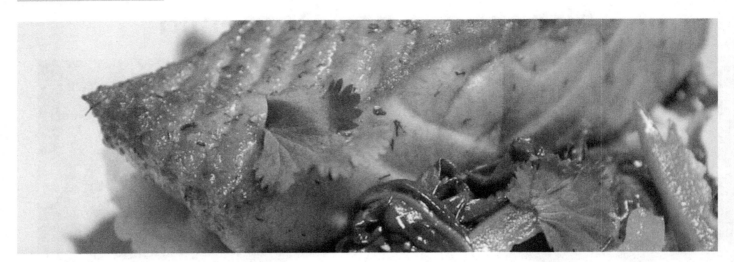

Ingredients

- 4 (6-ounce) salmon fillets
- 2 tablespoons extra-virgin olive oil
- Salt and freshly ground black pepper
- 2 bunches of asparagus, trimmed
- 2 cups cooked quinoa

Instructions

1. Preheat oven to 375°F.

2. Proceed by placing the salmon fillets on a baking sheet and brush each fillet with one teaspoon of olive oil, then season with salt and pepper.

3. Arrange asparagus around salmon and brush asparagus with the remaining olive oil.

4. Roast salmon and asparagus in preheated oven for 15 minutes.

5. Remove the baking sheet from the oven and top each salmon fillet with a portion of the cooked quinoa.

6. Return to oven and continue to bake for an additional 15 minutes.

7. Serve immediately.

Grilled Chicken Breast with Roasted Sweet Potatoes

Cook Time: 35 minutes

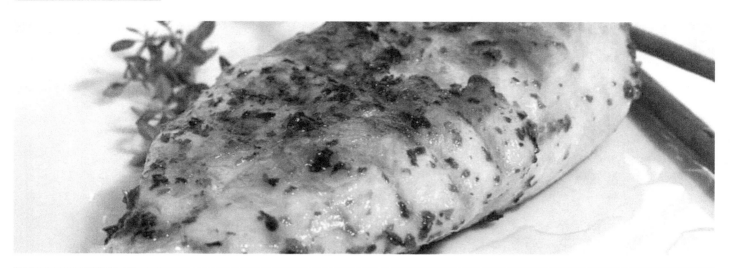

Ingredients

- 2 large sweet potatoes, cut into cubes
- 2 tablespoons olive oil
- Salt and pepper
- 2 boneless, skinless chicken breasts

Instructions

1. Preheat oven to 400°F.
2. On a baking sheet, place the sweet potatoes and drizzle with olive oil. Season with salt and pepper, then mix to combine.
3. Roast sweet potatoes in preheated oven for 20 minutes.
4. Heat a grill or grill pan to medium-high heat.
5. Season chicken breasts with salt and pepper and grill for 5 minutes per side.
6. Remove the baking sheet from the oven and add chicken breasts to the baking sheet with sweet potatoes.
7. Return to oven and continue to bake for an additional 10 minutes.
8. Serve chicken and sweet potatoes immediately.

Vegetable Soup with Lentils

Cook Time: 45 minutes

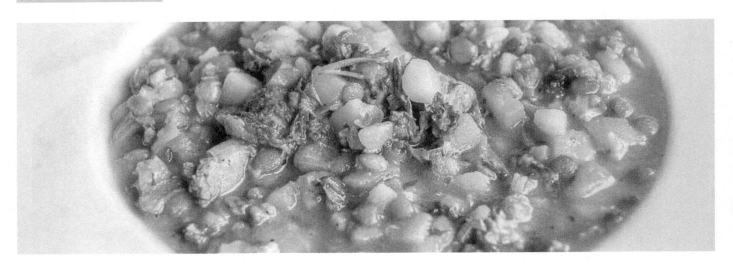

Ingredients

- 2 tablespoons olive oil
- 1 onion, diced
- 2 carrots, diced
- 2 stalks of celery, diced
- 2 cloves garlic, minced
- 1 teaspoon dried thyme
- 1 teaspoon dried oregano
- 6 cups vegetable broth
- 2 cups diced tomatoes
- 2 cups cooked lentils
- 2 cups spinach, chopped
- Salt and pepper

Instructions

1. Begin by heating olive oil in a large pot over medium heat.

2. Add onion, carrots, celery, garlic, thyme, and oregano. Cook, occasionally stirring for about 5 minutes, until vegetables are softened.

3. Add vegetable broth, tomatoes, and lentils. Boil, then proceed to reduce the heat and simmer for 20 minutes.

4. Add spinach and season with salt and pepper. Simmer for an additional 5 minutes.

5. Serve soup hot.

Cabbage and Bean Stew

Cook Time: 45 minutes

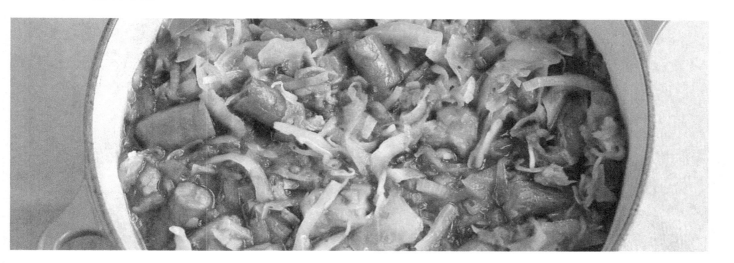

Ingredients

- 2 tablespoons olive oil
- 1 onion, diced
- 2 cloves garlic, minced
- 2 carrots, diced
- 1 teaspoon dried thyme
- 1 teaspoon dried oregano
- 2 cups shredded cabbage
- 1 (15-ounce) can of diced tomatoes
- 1 (15-ounce) can of rinsed and drained white beans
- 4 cups vegetable broth
- Salt and pepper

Instructions

1. Heat olive oil in a large pot over medium heat.

2. Add onion, garlic, carrots, thyme, and oregano. Cook, occasionally stirring for about 5 minutes, until vegetables are softened.

3. Add cabbage, tomatoes, beans, and vegetable broth. Boil, then reduce heat and simmer for 30 minutes.

4. Season with salt and pepper. Simmer for an additional 5 minutes.

5. Serve stew hot.

Broiled Trout with Brown Rice

Cook Time: 30 minutes

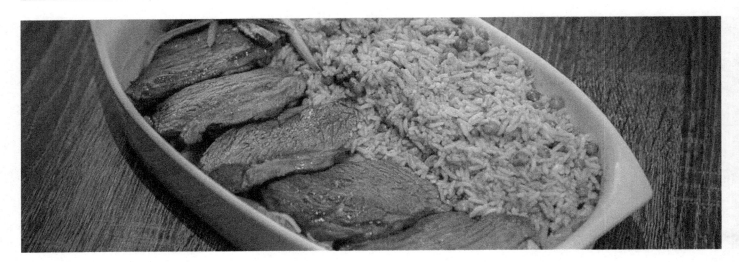

Ingredients

- 4 (6-ounce) trout fillets
- 2 tablespoons extra-virgin olive oil
- Salt and freshly ground black pepper
- 2 cups cooked brown rice

Instructions

1. Preheat the oven to broil.
2. Place the trout fillets on a baking sheet and brush each fillet with one teaspoon of olive oil, then season with salt and pepper.
3. Place baking sheet in preheated oven and broil for 10 minutes.
4. Remove the baking sheet from the oven and top each trout fillet with a portion of the cooked brown rice.
5. Return to oven and continue to broil for an additional 10 minutes.
6. Serve immediately.

Grilled Veggie and Feta Cheese Wrap

Cook Time: 25 minutes

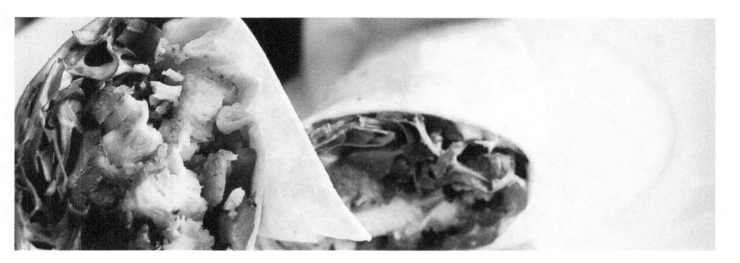

Ingredients

- 2 bell peppers, cut into strips
- 2 zucchini, cut into strips
- 2 tablespoons olive oil
- Salt and pepper
- 4 whole wheat tortillas
- 8 ounces feta cheese, crumbled

Instructions

1. Heat a grill or grill pan to medium-high heat.

2. Place bell peppers and zucchini in a large bowl and drizzle with olive oil. Season with salt and pepper, then mix to combine.

3. Grill vegetables for 5 minutes per side.

4. Place grilled vegetables on a plate and let cool slightly.

5. Place a tortilla on a work surface and top it with a portion of the grilled vegetables and feta cheese.

6. Roll up the tortilla and place it on a plate. Repeat with remaining tortillas.

7. Serve wraps immediately.

Quinoa and Kale Salad

Cook Time: 25 minutes

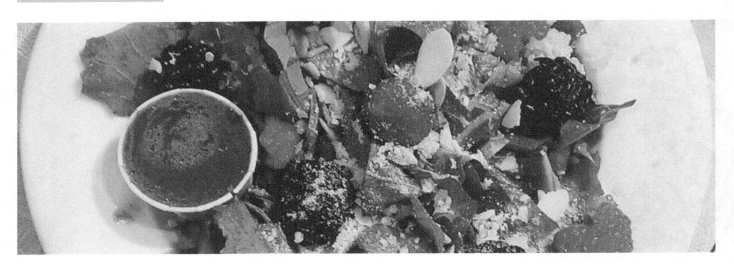

Ingredients

- 2 cups cooked quinoa
- 2 tablespoons extra-virgin olive oil
- 2 cloves garlic, minced
- 2 tablespoons lemon juice
- 2 tablespoons honey
- Salt and freshly ground black pepper
- 4 cups kale, chopped

Instructions

1. In a large bowl, combine quinoa, olive oil, garlic, lemon juice, honey, salt, and pepper. Mix to combine.
2. Add kale and toss to coat.
3. Serve salad immediately.

Baked Chicken with Roasted Vegetables

Cook Time: 45 minutes

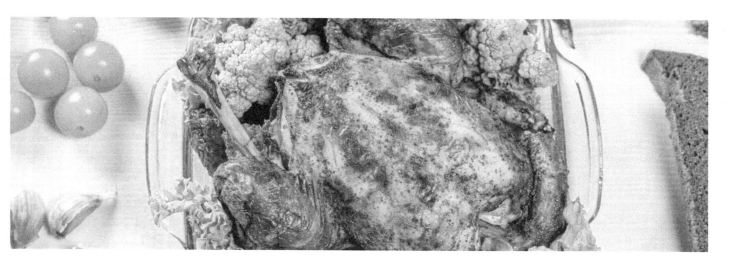

Ingredients

- 2 tablespoons olive oil
- 2 cloves garlic, minced
- 2 teaspoons paprika
- 2 teaspoons dried oregano
- 4 boneless, skinless chicken breasts
- 2 sweet potatoes, cut into cubes
- 2 bell peppers, cut into strips
- 2 zucchini, cut into strips
- Salt and pepper

Instructions

1. Preheat oven to 400°F.

2. In a large bowl, combine olive oil, garlic, paprika, oregano, and a pinch of salt and pepper.

3. Add chicken, sweet potatoes, bell peppers, and zucchini and mix to coat.

4. Arrange vegetables and chicken on a baking sheet and season with salt and pepper.

5. Roast in preheated oven for 30 minutes.

6. Serve chicken and vegetables immediately.

Spinach and Mushroom Omelet

Cook Time: 20 minutes

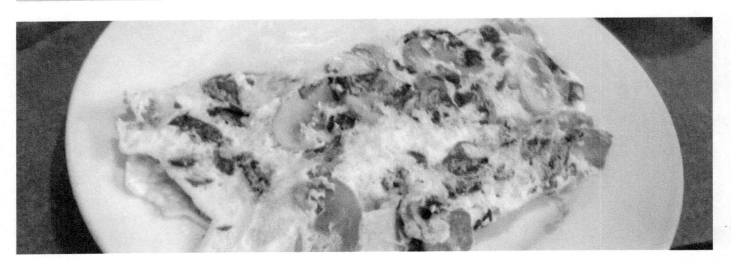

Ingredients

- 2 tablespoons olive oil
- 2 cloves garlic, minced
- 1 cup mushrooms, sliced
- 2 cups spinach, chopped
- 4 eggs
- 2 tablespoons milk
- Salt and pepper

Instructions

1. Heat olive oil in a medium skillet over medium heat.
2. Add garlic and mushrooms. Cook, occasionally stirring, until mushrooms are softened, about 5 minutes.
3. Add spinach and cook until wilted, about 2 minutes.
4. In a small bowl, whisk together eggs and milk. Season with salt and pepper.
5. Pour egg mixture into skillet and cook, stirring occasionally, until eggs are cooked through, about 5 minutes.
6. Serve the omelet hot.

Mediterranean Rice and Bean Bowl

Cook Time: 25 minutes

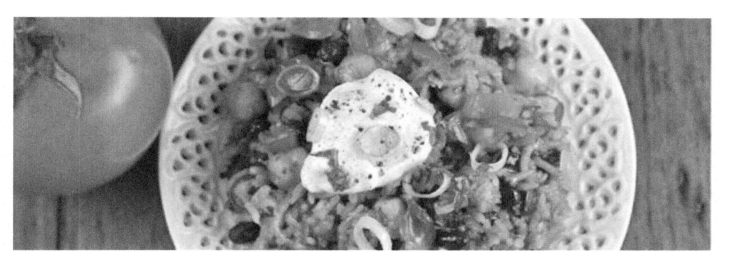

Ingredients

- 2 tablespoons olive oil
- 1 onion, diced
- 2 cloves garlic, minced
- 2 teaspoons paprika
- 2 teaspoons dried oregano
- 2 cups cooked rice
- 1 (15-ounce) can of white beans drained and rinsed
- 2 cups cherry tomatoes, halved
- 4 ounces feta cheese, crumbled
- Salt and pepper

Instructions

1. To begin, heat olive oil in a large skillet over medium heat.

2. Add onion, garlic, paprika, and oregano. Cook and stir occasionally, for about 5 minutes, until vegetables are softened.

3. Add cooked rice, beans, and tomatoes. Cook, occasionally stirring, for about 5 minutes until heated through.

4. Season with salt and pepper.

5. Divide mixture into four bowls and top with feta cheese.

6. Serve bowls immediately.

Turkey and Spinach Stuffed Peppers

Cook Time: 40 minutes

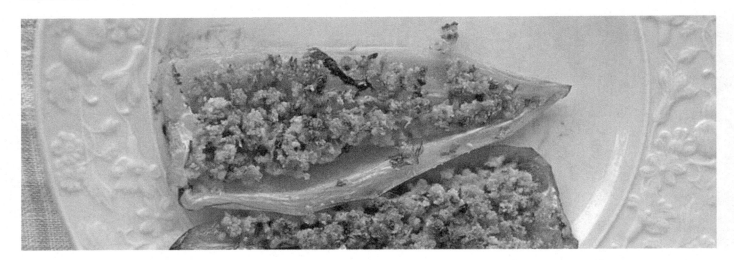

Ingredients

- 4 bell peppers
- 1 lb. ground turkey
- 1 onion, diced
- 2 cloves garlic, minced
- 1 tsp. olive oil
- 1 tsp. oregano
- 1 tsp. basil
- 1/2 tsp. paprika
- 1/2 tsp. thyme
- 1/4 tsp. cayenne pepper
- 1/4 tsp. salt
- 1/4 tsp. black pepper
- 2 cups fresh spinach leaves
- 1 cup cooked long-grain white rice
- 1/2 cup shredded mozzarella cheese

Instructions

1. Preheat oven to 375°F.

2. Cut bell peppers in half and remove seeds and membrane. Place in a baking dish.

3. Over medium-high heat, heat the olive oil in a large skillet. Add onion and garlic and sauté until softened, about 5 minutes.

4. Add ground turkey and seasonings to the skillet. Cook until turkey is browned, about 8 minutes.

5. Add spinach leaves to the skillet and cook until wilted, about 3 minutes.

6. Stir in cooked rice and remove from heat.

7. Fill each pepper half with turkey and spinach mixture and top with mozzarella cheese.

8. Bake for 25 minutes. Serve warm. Enjoy!

Steamed Fish and Vegetables

Cook Time: 15 minutes

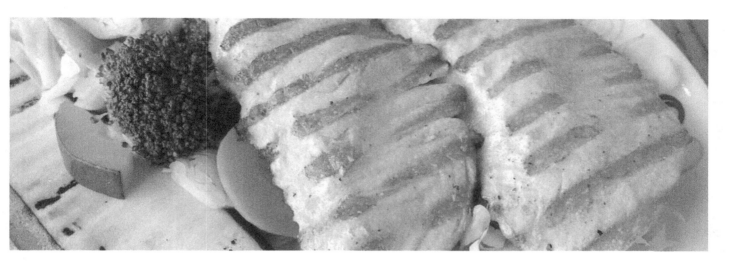

Ingredients

- 4 fillets of white fish (cod, haddock, etc.)
- 1 onion, sliced
- 1 red pepper, sliced
- 1 zucchini, sliced
- 1 bell pepper, sliced
- 1/2 cup white wine
- 1/4 cup vegetable broth
- 2 cloves garlic, minced
- 1 tsp. olive oil
- 1/2 tsp. oregano
- 1/2 tsp. thyme
- 1/2 tsp. basil
- 1/4 tsp. salt
- 1/4 tsp. black pepper

Instructions

1. In a large steamer pot, add enough water to reach the bottom of the steamer basket. Place the steamer basket in the pot and bring it to a boil.

2. Place onion, red pepper, zucchini, and bell pepper in the steamer basket.

3. Place the fish fillets on top of the vegetables and sprinkle them with garlic, oregano, thyme, basil, salt, and pepper.

4. Drizzle the fish and vegetables with olive oil and white wine.

5. Place a lid on the steamer pot and steam for 10-15 minutes or until the fish is cooked through.

6. Serve warm. Enjoy!

Roasted Vegetable and Farro Salad

Cook Time: 25 minutes

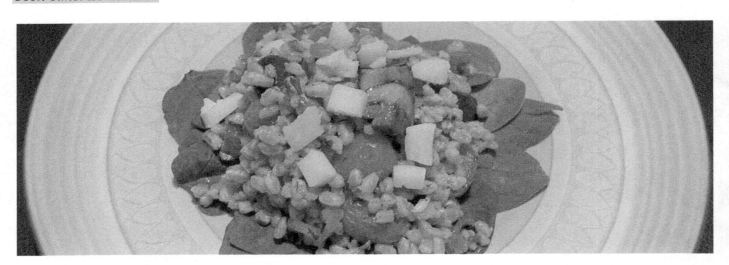

Ingredients

- 1/2 cup farro
- 1 zucchini, diced
- 1 yellow squash, diced
- 1 red bell pepper, diced
- 1/2 red onion, diced
- 2 cloves garlic, minced
- 2 tsp. olive oil
- 1/2 tsp. oregano
- 1/4 tsp. salt
- 1/4 tsp. black pepper
- 1/4 cup crumbled feta cheese
- 1/4 cup pitted Kalamata olives

Instructions

1. Preheat oven to 375°F.

2. In a medium pot, bring 1 cup of water to a boil. Add farro and cook until tender, about 20 minutes. Drain and set aside.

3. In a large bowl, combine zucchini, yellow squash, bell pepper, onion, garlic, olive oil, oregano, salt, and pepper.

4. Place vegetables on a baking sheet and roast in the preheated oven for 20 minutes, stirring halfway through.

5. In a large bowl, combine cooked farro, roasted vegetables, feta cheese, and olives.

6. Serve warm or chilled. Enjoy!

Baked Halibut with Rice Pilaf

Cook Time: 25 minutes

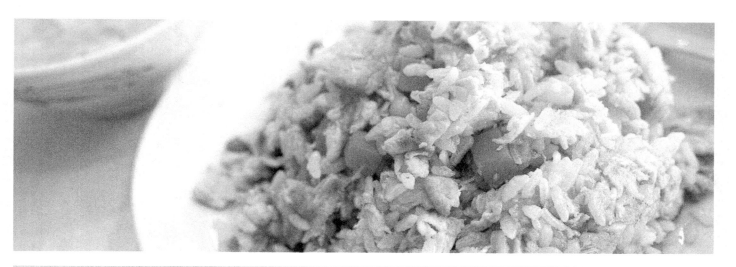

Ingredients

- 4 fillets of halibut
- 1 cup long-grain white rice
- 2 cups vegetable broth
- 1/4 cup olive oil
- 1 onion, diced
- 1 red bell pepper, diced
- 2 cloves garlic, minced
- 1 tsp. oregano
- 1/2 tsp. thyme
- 1/4 tsp. salt
- 1/4 tsp. black pepper
- 1/4 cup fresh parsley, chopped

Instructions

1. Preheat oven to 375°F.

2. In a medium pot, bring vegetable broth to a boil. Add rice and reduce heat to low. Simmer until rice is tender, about 15 minutes.

3. Over medium-high heat, heat the olive oil in a large skillet. Add onion, bell pepper, and garlic and sauté until softened, about 5 minutes.

4. Add oregano, thyme, salt, and pepper to the skillet and mix to combine.

5. Place halibut fillets in a baking dish and top with the onion and bell pepper mixture.

6. Bake for 15 minutes or until halibut is cooked through.

7. Serve halibut with cooked rice pilaf and top with fresh parsley. Enjoy!

Roasted Tomato and Basil Soup

Cook Time: 45 minutes

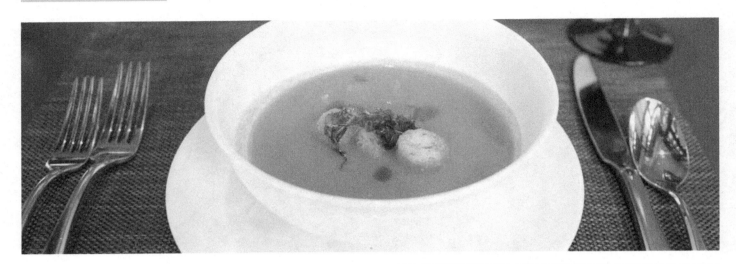

Ingredients

- 5 large tomatoes, chopped
- 1 onion, diced
- 2 cloves garlic, minced
- 2 tsp. olive oil
- 1/2 tsp. oregano
- 1/4 tsp. thyme
- 1/4 tsp. salt
- 1/4 tsp. black pepper
- 2 cups vegetable broth
- 1/4 cup heavy cream
- 1/4 cup fresh basil, chopped

Instructions

1. Preheat oven to 375°F.

2. Place tomatoes, onion, and garlic on a baking sheet. Drizzle with olive oil and season with oregano, thyme, salt, and pepper. Roast in the preheated oven for 30 minutes.

3. Transfer roasted vegetables to a large pot and add vegetable broth. Boil, then proceed by reducing heat to low, and simmer for 10 minutes.

4. Using an immersion blender, blend soup until smooth.

5. Stir in heavy cream and fresh basil and simmer for an additional 5 minutes.

6. Serve warm. Enjoy!

Greek-Style Chicken with Spinach

Cook Time: 30 minutes

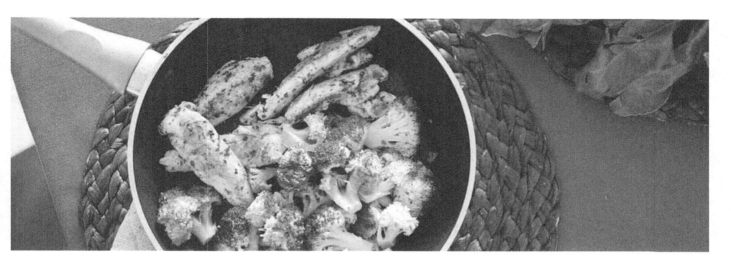

Ingredients

- 4 boneless, skinless chicken breasts
- 1 onion, diced
- 2 cloves garlic, minced
- 1 tsp. olive oil
- 1/2 tsp. oregano
- 1/2 tsp. thyme
- 1/2 tsp. Rosemary
- 1/4 tsp. salt
- 1/4 tsp. black pepper
- 1/2 cup crumbled feta cheese
- 2 cups fresh spinach leaves
- 1/4 cup pitted Kalamata olives

Instructions

1. Preheat oven to 375°F.
2. Over medium-high heat, heat the olive oil in a large skillet. Add onion and garlic and sauté until softened, about 5 minutes.
3. Place chicken breasts in a baking dish and season with oregano, thyme, rosemary, salt, and pepper. Top with onion and garlic mixture.
4. Bake for 20 minutes or until chicken is cooked through.
5. Top chicken with feta cheese, spinach leaves, and Kalamata olives.
6. Bake for an additional 5 minutes or until the cheese is melted.
7. Serve warm. Enjoy!

Grilled Haloumi Cheese with Zucchini

Cook Time: 10 minutes

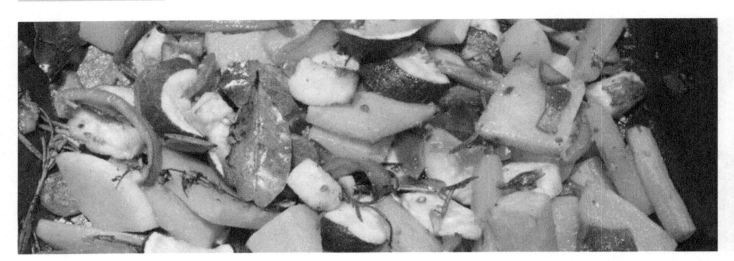

Ingredients

- 1/2 lb. haloumi cheese
- 1 zucchini, sliced
- 1 tsp. olive oil
- 1/2 tsp. oregano
- 1/4 tsp. salt
- 1/4 tsp. black pepper

Instructions

1. Begin by heating a large non-stick skillet over medium-high heat.
2. Slice halloumi cheese into 1/4-inch slices.
3. Drizzle zucchini with olive oil, oregano, salt, and pepper.
4. Place zucchini slices in the hot skillet and cook for 2 minutes.
5. Add halloumi cheese slices and cook for 2 minutes. Flip and cook for an additional 2 minutes or until the cheese is golden brown.
6. Serve warm. Enjoy!

Chickpea and Spinach Curry

Cook Time: 25 minutes

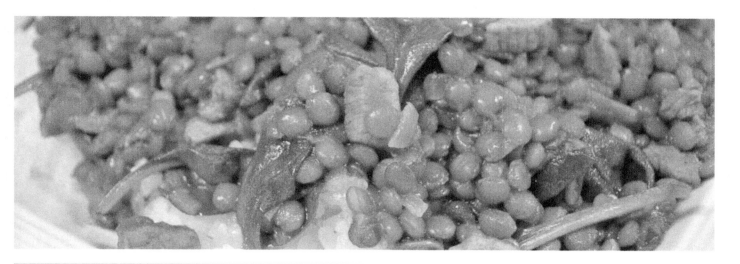

Ingredients

- 1 can chickpeas, drained and rinsed
- 1 onion, diced
- 2 cloves garlic, minced
- 2 tsp. olive oil
- 1 can (14 oz.) diced tomatoes
- 2 tsp. curry powder
- 1/4 tsp. cumin
- 1/4 tsp. salt
- 1/4 tsp. black pepper
- 2 cups fresh spinach leaves

Instructions

1. In a large skillet over medium-high heat, heat olive oil. Add onion and garlic and sauté until softened, about 5 minutes.

2. Add diced tomatoes, curry powder, cumin, salt, and pepper to the skillet and mix to combine.

3. Add chickpeas and spinach leaves to the skillet and cook until spinach is wilted about 5 minutes.

4. Serve warm. Enjoy!

Mediterranean Chickpea Salad

Cook Time: 10 minutes

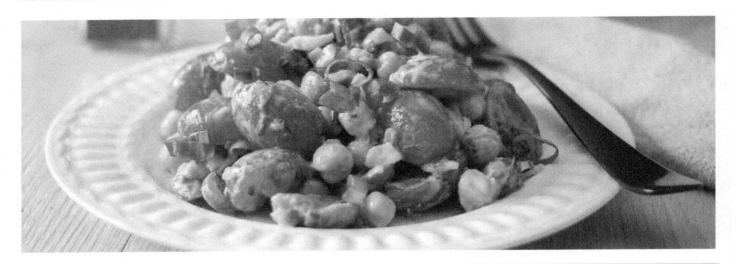

Ingredients

- 1 can chickpeas, drained and rinsed
- 1/4 cup red onion, diced
- 1/4 cup crumbled feta cheese
- 1/4 cup pitted Kalamata olives
- 1/4 cup fresh parsley, chopped
- 1 tsp. olive oil
- 1 tsp. red wine vinegar
- 1/4 tsp. oregano
- 1/4 tsp. salt
- 1/4 tsp. black pepper

Instructions

1. In a large bowl, combine chickpeas, red onion, feta cheese, Kalamata olives, and parsley.

2. In a small bowl, whisk together olive oil, red wine vinegar, oregano, salt, and pepper.

3. Pour dressing over chickpea salad and mix to combine.

4. Serve chilled. Enjoy!

Turkey and Black Bean Chili

Cook Time: 1hr 10 minutes

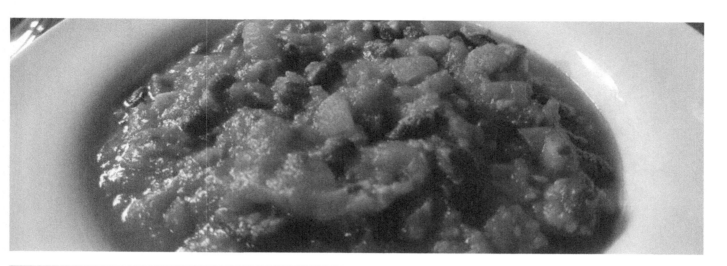

Ingredients

- 1 lb. ground turkey
- 2 garlic cloves, minced
- 1 onion, chopped
- 1 bell pepper, chopped
- 2 cans (15 oz each) of black beans, rinsed and drained
- 1 can (14.5 oz) diced tomatoes
- 2 tablespoons chili powder
- 1 teaspoon ground cumin
- 1 teaspoon dried oregano
- ¼ teaspoon ground black pepper
- 2 cups chicken broth

Instructions

1. Over medium-high heat, heat a large saucepan

2. Add turkey, garlic, onion, and bell pepper; cook, stirring and breaking up the turkey until the turkey is cooked through about 8 minutes.

3. Add beans, tomatoes, chili powder, cumin, oregano, pepper, and broth; bring to a boil.

4. Reduce heat to low and simmer, uncovered, for 1 hour.

5. Serve chili hot.

Lentil and Veggie Stuffed Peppers

Cook Time: 1hr 10 minutes

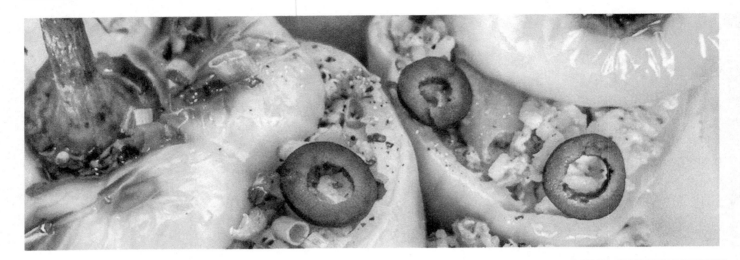

Ingredients

- 1 cup dry green lentils
- 4 bell peppers (any color)
- 1 onion, chopped
- 2 cloves garlic, minced
- 1 tablespoon olive oil
- 1 can (14.5 oz) diced tomatoes
- 1 teaspoon dried oregano
- 1 teaspoon ground cumin
- ½ teaspoon ground black pepper
- 1 cup shredded cheese

Instructions

1. Preheat oven to 350°F.
2. In a large saucepan, bring 2 cups of water to a boil.
3. Add lentils and reduce heat to low. Simmer, uncovered, for 15 minutes. Drain and set aside.
4. Cut the tops off the bell peppers and remove the seeds and ribs.
5. In a large skillet, heat oil over medium heat.
6. Add onion and garlic; cook, stirring, until softened, about 5 minutes.
7. Add tomatoes, oregano, cumin, and pepper; cook, stirring, for 2 minutes.
8. Add lentils and cook, stirring, for 1 minute. Remove from heat.
9. Fill each pepper with the lentil mixture and top with cheese.
10. Place peppers in a baking dish and bake for 45 minutes.

Baked Eggplant Parmesan

Cook Time: 1hr 10 minutes

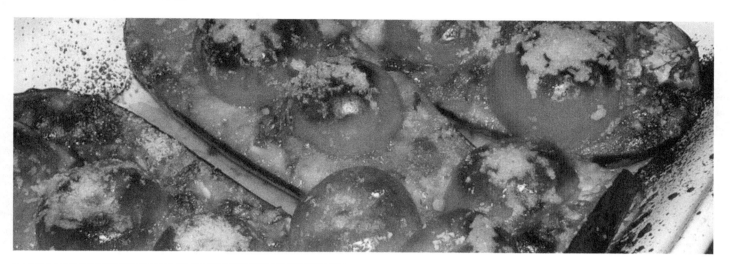

Ingredients

- 2 large eggplants, sliced into ½-inch rounds
- 2 tablespoons olive oil
- 1 teaspoon salt
- 1 teaspoon black pepper
- 2 cups marinara sauce
- 1 cup shredded mozzarella cheese
- ¼ cup grated Parmesan cheese

Instructions

1. Preheat oven to 375°F.
2. Place eggplant slices on a baking sheet. Sprinkle with olive oil and season with salt and pepper.
3. Bake for 25 minutes, flipping halfway through.
4. Spread ½ cup of marinara sauce in the bottom of a 9x13-inch baking dish.
5. Layer half of the eggplant slices in the dish, followed by a layer of marinara sauce.
6. Sprinkle with ½ cup of mozzarella cheese and 2 tablespoons of Parmesan cheese.
7. Repeat with the remaining eggplant, marinara sauce, and cheese.
8. Bake for 25 minutes or until cheese is melted and bubbly.

Broiled Halibut with Lemon and Tomatoes

Cook Time: 20 minutes

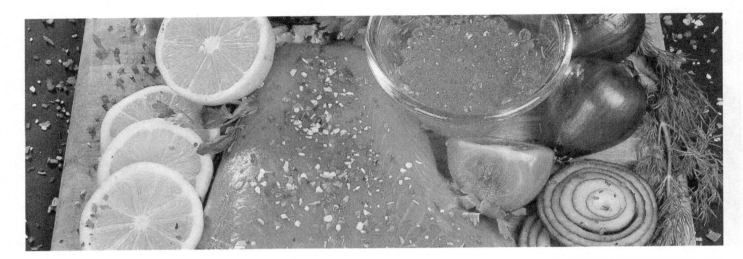

Ingredients

- 2 tablespoons olive oil
- 2 cloves garlic, minced
- 2 tablespoons chopped fresh parsley
- 2 tablespoons fresh lemon juice
- 1 teaspoon dried oregano
- 1 teaspoon salt
- ½ teaspoon black pepper
- 2 halibut fillets (about 6 oz each)
- 2 Roma tomatoes, chopped

Instructions

1. Preheat the broiler.
2. In a small bowl, combine oil, garlic, parsley, lemon juice, oregano, salt, and pepper.
3. Place halibut in a broiler-safe baking dish. Brush with the oil mixture.
4. Top with tomatoes.
5. Broil for 8 minutes, or until the fish is cooked through.

Zucchini and Roasted Red Pepper Frittata

Cook Time: 45 minutes

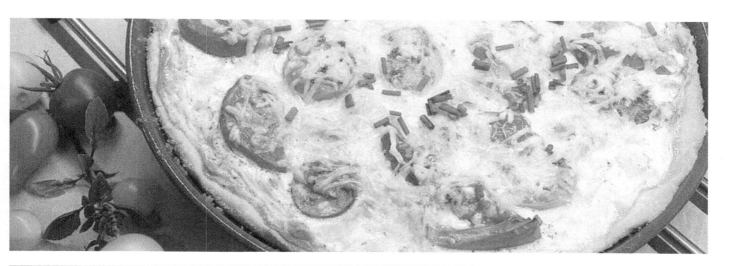

Ingredients

- 2 tablespoons olive oil
- 1 onion, chopped
- 2 cloves garlic, minced
- 2 zucchini, sliced
- 1 roasted red pepper, chopped
- 6 large eggs
- ½ cup grated Parmesan cheese
- Salt and black pepper, to taste

Instructions

1. Preheat oven to 375°F.
2. Proceed by heating oil in a large ovenproof skillet over medium heat.
3. Add onion and garlic; cook, stirring, until softened, about 5 minutes.
4. Add zucchini and red pepper; cook, stirring, for 3 minutes.
5. In a medium bowl, whisk together eggs, Parmesan cheese, salt, and pepper.
6. Pour egg mixture into the skillet.
7. Cook until the edges are set, about 5 minutes.
8. Place the skillet in the oven and bake for 20 minutes or until the center is set.

Grilled Vegetable and Quinoa Salad

Cook Time: 40 minutes

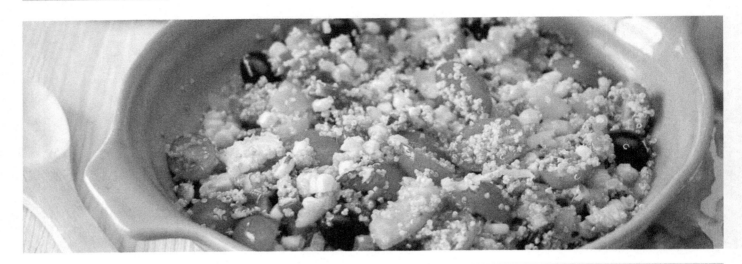

Ingredients

- 2 tablespoons olive oil
- 1 red bell pepper, chopped
- 1 yellow bell pepper, chopped
- 1 zucchini, sliced
- 1 onion, sliced
- 2 cloves garlic, minced
- 2 cups cooked quinoa
- ¼ cup chopped fresh parsley
- 2 tablespoons red wine vinegar
- Salt and black pepper, to taste

Instructions

1. Preheat a grill to medium-high heat.

2. In a medium bowl, combine oil, bell peppers, zucchini, onion, and garlic; toss to coat.

3. Place vegetables on the grill and cook for 10 minutes, flipping halfway through.

4. In a large bowl, combine cooked vegetables, quinoa, parsley, vinegar, salt, and pepper.

5. Toss to combine and serve.

Baked Salmon with Spinach

Cook Time: 25 minutes

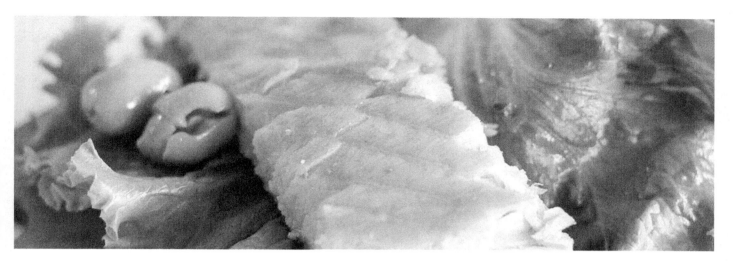

Ingredients

- 2 tablespoons olive oil
- 4 salmon fillets (6 oz each)
- 2 cloves garlic, minced
- 2 cups baby spinach
- ½ cup sun-dried tomatoes, chopped
- ¼ cup grated Parmesan cheese
- Salt and black pepper, to taste

Instructions

1. Preheat oven to 350°F.
2. Proceed by heating oil in a large ovenproof skillet over medium heat.
3. Add salmon and garlic; cook for 3 minutes.
4. Flip salmon and cook for 3 minutes.
5. Add spinach and sun-dried tomatoes; cook for 2 minutes.
6. Sprinkle Parmesan cheese over the top.
7. Place skillet in the oven and bake for 12 minutes, or until salmon is cooked through.

Shrimp and Vegetable Stir Fry

Cook Time: 20 minutes

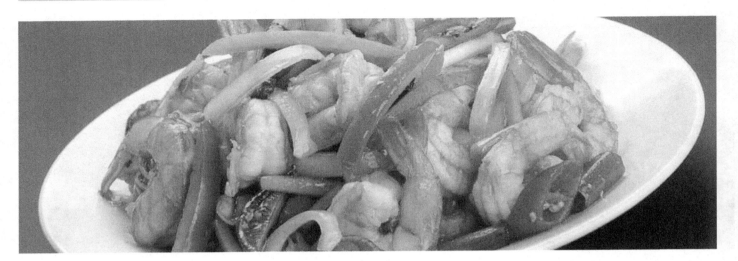

Ingredients

- 2 tablespoons vegetable oil
- 1 onion, chopped
- 1 bell pepper, chopped
- 2 cloves garlic, minced
- 1 cup sliced mushrooms
- 1 cup snow peas
- 1 lb. medium shrimp, peeled and deveined
- 2 tablespoons soy sauce
- 2 tablespoons sesame oil
- 2 tablespoons rice vinegar
- 2 teaspoons sugar
- 2 tablespoons chopped fresh cilantro

Instructions

1. Heat oil in a large skillet or wok over medium-high heat.

2. Add onion, bell pepper, garlic, mushrooms, and snow peas; cook, stirring, for 5 minutes.

3. Add shrimp; cook, stirring, for 2 minutes.

4. Add soy sauce, sesame oil, vinegar, and sugar; cook, stirring, for 2 minutes.

5. Stir in cilantro and serve.

Roasted Vegetable and Feta Cheese Wrap

Cook Time: 30 minutes

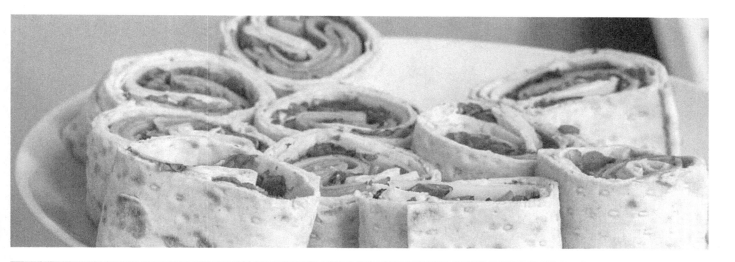

Ingredients

- 2 tablespoons olive oil
- 1 red bell pepper, chopped
- 1 yellow bell pepper, chopped
- 1 zucchini, sliced
- 1 onion, sliced
- 2 cloves garlic, minced
- 4 large flour tortillas
- ½ cup crumbled feta cheese
- Salt and black pepper, to taste

Instructions

1. Preheat oven to 400°F.
2. In a medium bowl, combine oil, bell peppers, zucchini, onion, and garlic; toss to coat.
3. Place vegetables on a baking sheet and roast for 25 minutes, or until tender.
4. Divide vegetables among the tortillas and top with feta cheese.
5. Season with salt and pepper, to taste.
6. Fold the tortillas and serve.

Baked Salmon with Lemon-Herb Sauce

Cook Time: 25 minutes

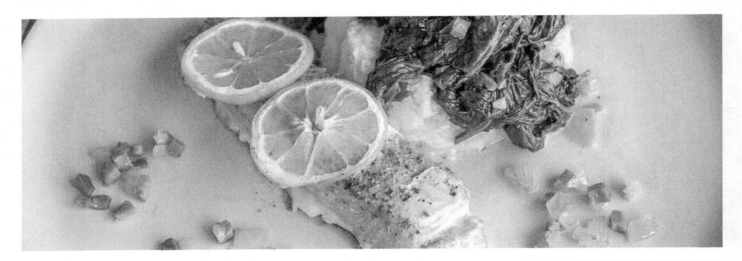

Ingredients

- 2 tablespoons olive oil
- 4 salmon fillets (6 oz each)
- 1 tablespoon lemon juice
- 2 cloves garlic, minced
- 2 tablespoons chopped fresh parsley
- 2 tablespoons chopped fresh basil
- Salt and black pepper, to taste

Instructions

1. Preheat oven to 350°F.
2. Proceed by heating oil in a large ovenproof skillet over medium heat.
3. Add salmon and garlic; cook for 3 minutes.
4. Flip salmon and cook for 3 minutes.
5. Add lemon juice, parsley, and basil; cook for 1 minute.
6. Place skillet in the oven and bake for 12 minutes, or until salmon is cooked through.
7. Season with salt and pepper to taste.

Snack Recipes for the Mind Diet for Alzheimer's and Dementia

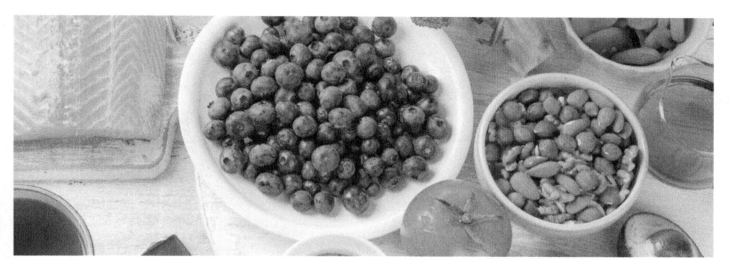

Snacking is an important part of any healthy diet, and it can be particularly important for individuals with Alzheimer's and dementia. Snacks can help maintain energy levels throughout the day and prevent overeating at mealtime. When it comes to the Mind Diet for Alzheimer's and dementia, there are several snack recipes that can support brain health.

Some snack options for the Mind Diet include nuts, seeds, and dried fruit, which are high in healthy fats and antioxidants. Hummus with raw vegetables, such as carrots or celery, is another great option as it provides fiber and protein while being low in saturated fat. Greek yogurt with fresh berries is another tasty snack that is high in protein and calcium.

If you're looking for something sweet, try making fruit smoothies or energy balls made with dates, nuts, and dark chocolate. These snacks are rich in antioxidants and can satisfy a sweet tooth while also providing important nutrients for brain health.

Avocado Toast with Sprouted Whole-Grain Bread

Cook Time: 5 minutes

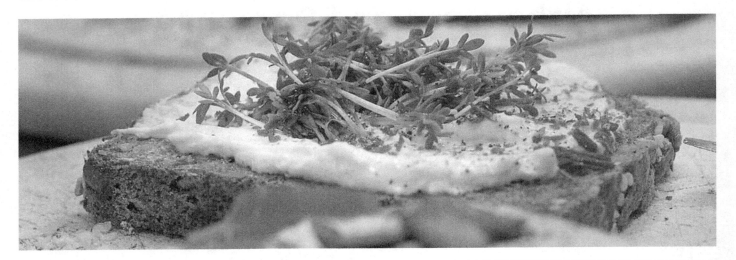

Ingredients

- 1 slice of sprouted whole-grain bread
- 1/2 avocado, mashed
- 1/2 teaspoon olive oil
- Salt and pepper to taste

Instructions

1. Toast the sprouted whole-grain bread.
2. Mash the avocado and mix in the olive oil in a small bowl.
3. Spread the avocado mixture onto the toasted bread.
4. Sprinkle with salt and pepper.
5. Enjoy!

Roasted Chickpeas

Prep Time: 10 minutes

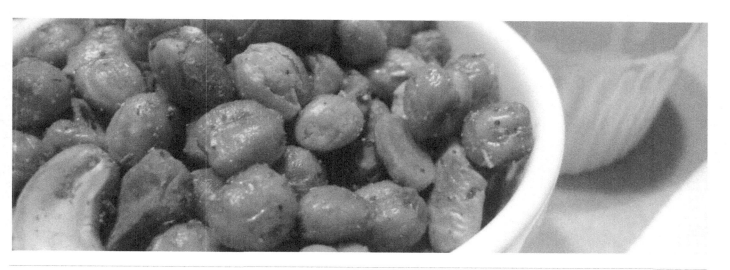

Ingredients

- 1 can chickpeas, drained and rinsed
- 1 tablespoon olive oil
- 1 teaspoon garlic powder
- 1 teaspoon smoked paprika
- 1/4 teaspoon sea salt

Instructions

1. Preheat oven to 400°F.
2. Drain and rinse the chickpeas and pat dry with a paper towel.
3. In a bowl, mix together the olive oil, garlic powder, smoked paprika, and sea salt.
4. Toss the chickpeas in the mixture until they are evenly coated.
5. Spread the chickpeas on a baking sheet and roast in the oven for 20-25 minutes or until golden and crispy.
6. Enjoy!

Apple Slices with Almond Butter

Prep Time: 5 minutes

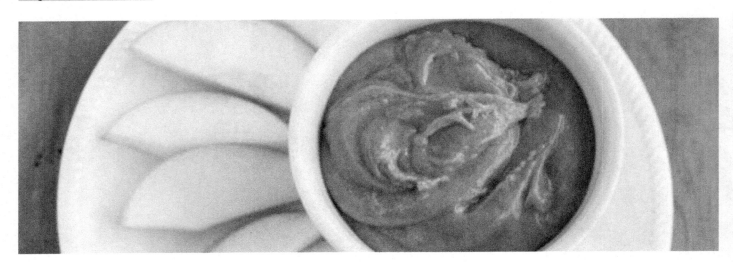

Ingredients

- 2 apples, thinly sliced
- 2 tablespoon almond butter

Instructions

1. Thinly slice the apples.
2. Spread the almond butter over the apple slices.
3. Enjoy!

Greek Yogurt with Berries

Prep Time: 5 minutes

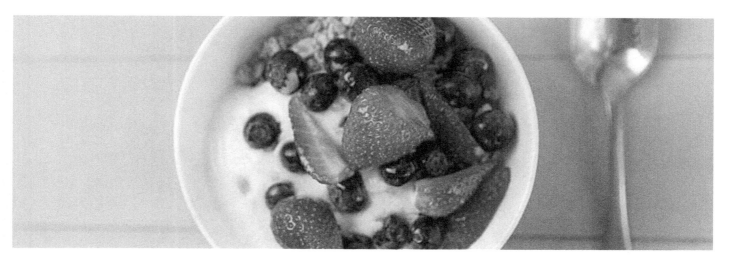

Ingredients

- 1 cup Greek yogurt
- 1/2 cup fresh or frozen berries

Instructions

1. Place the Greek yogurt in a bowl.
2. Top with fresh or frozen berries.
3. Enjoy!

Trail Mix with Nuts and Dried Fruit

Prep Time: 5 minutes

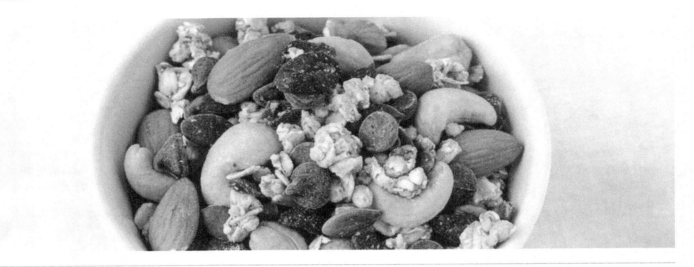

Ingredients

- 1/2 cup nuts (almonds, walnuts, pecans, etc.)
- 1/4 cup dried fruit (raisins, cranberries, dates, etc.)

Instructions

1. In a bowl, mix together the nuts and dried fruit.
2. Enjoy!

Roasted Veggies with Hummus

Prep Time: 20 minutes

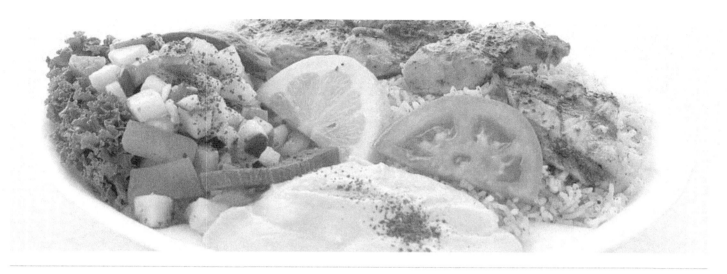

Ingredients

- 1 cup diced vegetables (carrots, bell peppers, onions, etc.)
- 1 tablespoon olive oil
- Salt and pepper to taste
- 1/2 cup hummus

Instructions

1. Preheat oven to 400°F.
2. In a bowl, mix together the diced vegetables, olive oil, salt, and pepper.
3. Spread the vegetables on a baking sheet and roast in the oven for 10-15 minutes or until golden and tender.
4. Serve the roasted vegetables with hummus.
5. Enjoy!

Kale Chips

Prep Time: 15 minutes

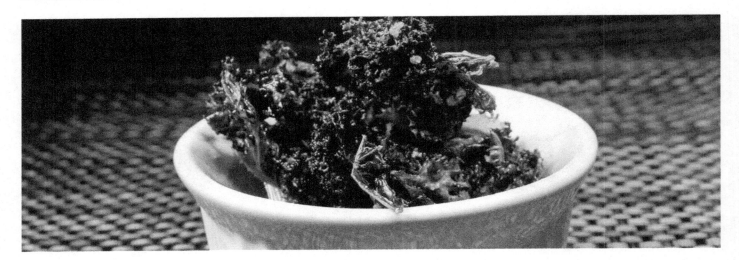

Ingredients

- 1 bunch of kale
- 1 tablespoon olive oil
- Salt and pepper to taste

Instructions

1. Preheat oven to 375°F.
2. Rinse and pat dry the kale.
3. Cut off the stems and tear the leaves into bite-sized pieces.
4. In a bowl, mix together the kale, olive oil, salt, and pepper.
5. Spread the kale on a baking sheet and bake in the oven for 10-15 minutes or until crisp and lightly browned.
6. Enjoy!

Blueberry and Oat Smoothie

Prep Time: 5 minutes

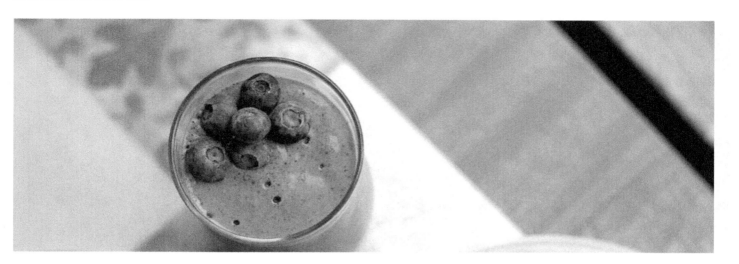

Ingredients

- 1/2 cup frozen blueberries
- 1/2 cup plain Greek yogurt
- 1/4 cup rolled oats
- 1 cup almond milk

Instructions

1. Place the frozen blueberries, Greek yogurt, rolled oats, and almond milk in a blender.
2. Blend until smooth.
3. Enjoy!

Dark Chocolate with Almonds

Prep Time: 5 minutes

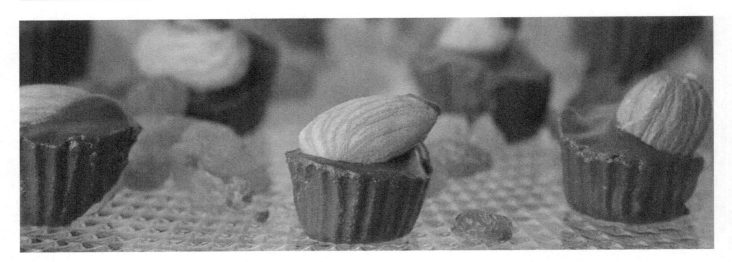

Ingredients

- 1/4 cup dark chocolate chips
- 1/4 cup sliced almonds

Instructions

1. Place the dark chocolate chips in a microwave-safe bowl.
2. Microwave for 30 seconds, then stir.
3. Continue to microwave in 30-second intervals until the chocolate is melted.
4. Stir in the sliced almonds.
5. Pour the mixture onto a parchment paper-lined baking sheet and spread it into an even layer.
6. Place in the fridge to cool.
7. Break into pieces and enjoy!

Edamame

Prep Time: 5 minutes *Cook Time: 10 minutes*

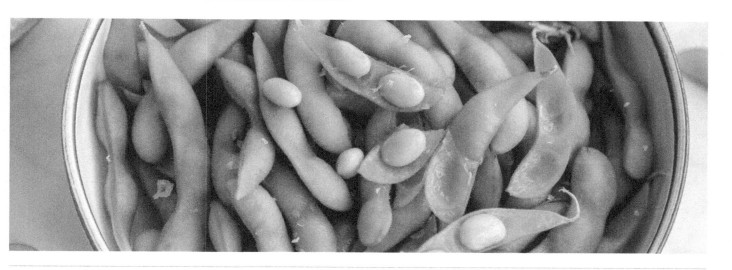

Ingredients

- 1 lb. of frozen edamame
- 1 teaspoon of salt

Instructions

1. Put a cup of water in a pot and bring to boil.
2. Add the edamame and salt to the boiling water and stir.
3. Boil the edamame for 8-10 minutes or until it's cooked through.
4. Strain the edamame and serve with a sprinkle of salt.

Overnight Oats

Prep Time: 5 minutes *Cook Time: 0 minutes*

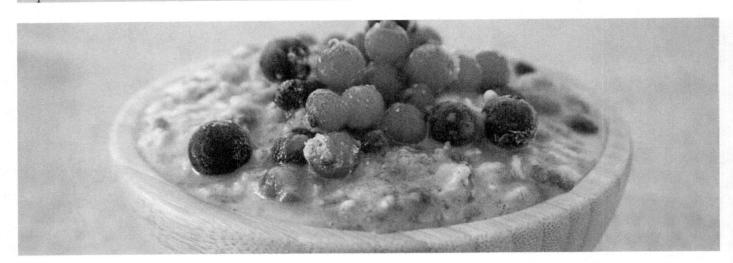

Ingredients

- 1 cup of rolled oats
- 1 cup of milk
- 1 teaspoon of honey
- 1/2 teaspoon of cinnamon
- 1/4 cup of raisins (optional)

Instructions

1. Mix together the oats, milk, honey, and cinnamon in a bowl.
2. Add in the raisins, if desired.
3. Stir until everything is combined.
4. Cover the bowl and put it in the refrigerator overnight.
5. Serve the oats cold the next morning.

Cottage Cheese with Fruit

Prep Time: 5 minutes   *Cook Time: 0 minutes*

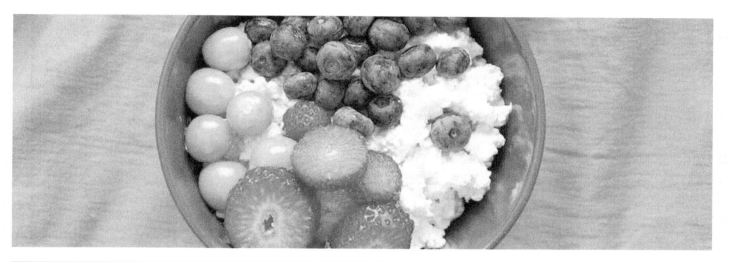

Ingredients

- 1 cup of cottage cheese
- 1/2 cup of diced fresh fruit (such as strawberries, blueberries, or bananas)

Instructions

1. In a bowl, mix together the cottage cheese and fruit.
2. Serve the mixture cold or at room temperature.

Pumpkin Seeds

Prep Time: 5 minutes *Cook Time: 15 minutes*

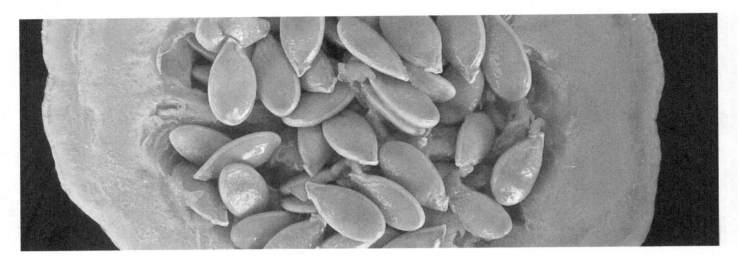

Ingredients

- 1 cup of raw pumpkin seeds
- 1 teaspoon of olive oil
- 1/2 teaspoon of salt

Instructions

1. To begin, preheat the oven to 350 degrees Fahrenheit.
2. Spread the pumpkin seeds out on a parchment-lined baking sheet.
3. Drizzle the olive oil over the seeds and sprinkle with the salt.
4. Bake for 12-15 minutes, stirring once halfway through the baking time.
5. Serve the pumpkin seeds warm or at room temperature.

Cauliflower Tots

Prep Time: 15 minutes   *Cook Time: 25 minutes*

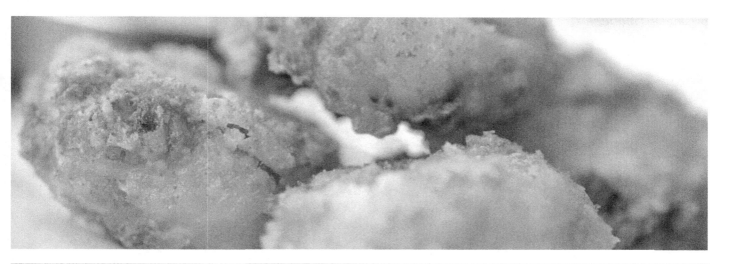

Ingredients

- 1 head of cauliflower, cut into florets
- 1/4 cup of flour
- 1/4 cup of grated Parmesan cheese
- 2 tablespoons of chopped parsley
- 1/2 teaspoon of garlic powder
- 1/4 teaspoon of salt
- 1/4 teaspoon of black pepper
- 1 egg, lightly beaten

Instructions

1. To begin, preheat the oven to 375 degrees Fahrenheit.
2. Place the cauliflower florets in a food processor and pulse until it is finely chopped.
3. Transfer the cauliflower to a bowl and add the flour, Parmesan cheese, parsley, garlic powder, salt, and pepper.
4. Stir in the egg until everything is combined.
5. Form the mixture into small tots and place them on a parchment-lined baking sheet.
6. Bake for 20-25 minutes or until the tots are golden brown.
7. Serve the tots warm.

Fruit and Nut Bars

Prep Time: 10 minutes   *Cook Time: 25 minutes*

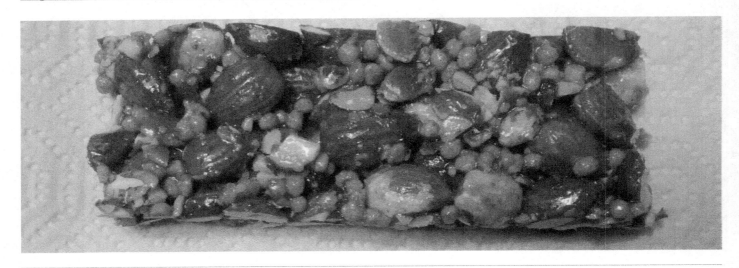

Ingredients

- 1/2 cup of rolled oats
- 1/2 cup of chopped nuts (such as almonds, walnuts, or pecans)
- 1/4 cup of honey
- 1/4 cup of dried fruit (such as raisins, cranberries, or dates)

Instructions

1. To begin, preheat the oven to 350 degrees Fahrenheit.
2. In a bowl, mix together the oats, nuts, honey, and dried fruit.
3. Spread the mixture out on a parchment-lined baking sheet.
4. Bake for 20-25 minutes or until the mixture is lightly browned.
5. Let the bars cool before cutting them into bars.
6. Serve the bars at room temperature.

Hummus and Veggie Wraps

Prep Time: 10 minutes   *Cook Time: 0 minutes*

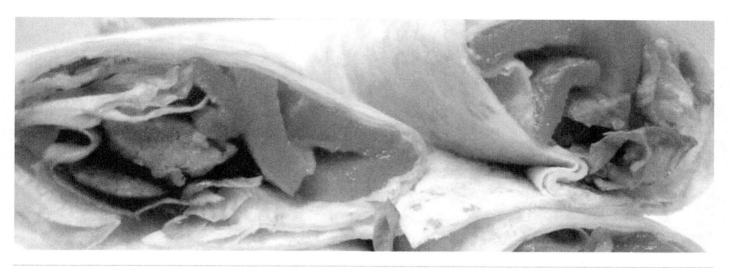

Ingredients

- 1 whole wheat wrap
- 1/4 cup of hummus
- 1/4 cup of diced raw vegetables (such as tomatoes, cucumbers, and bell peppers)

Instructions

1. Spread the hummus on the wrap.
2. Add the diced vegetables on top of the hummus.
3. Roll the wrap-up and cut it in half.
4. Serve the wrap cold or at room temperature.

Popcorn with Olive Oil

Prep Time: 5 minutes   *Cook Time:* 5 minutes

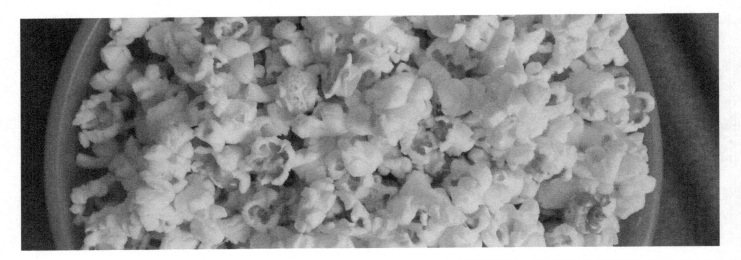

Ingredients

- 1/4 cup of popcorn kernels
- 1 tablespoon of olive oil
- 1 teaspoon of salt (optional)

Instructions

1. To begin, heat the olive oil in a large saucepan over medium heat.
2. Add the popcorn kernels to the pan and cover it with a lid.
3. Shake the pan occasionally to prevent the kernels from burning.
4. When the kernels have stopped popping, remove the pan from the heat.
5. Sprinkle with salt, if desired, and serve the popcorn warm.

Quinoa and Black Bean Salad

Prep Time: 10 minutes   *Cook Time: 20 minutes*

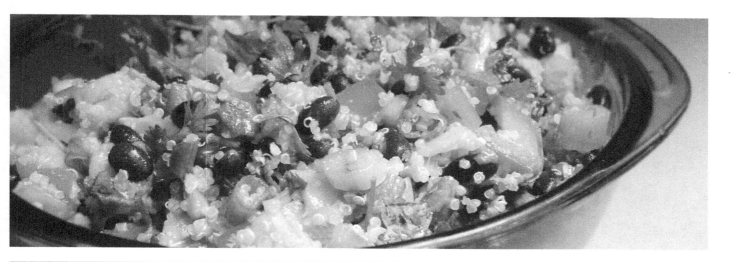

Ingredients

- 1 cup of quinoa
- 1/2 cup of cooked black beans
- 1/4 cup of diced red onions
- 1/4 cup of diced red bell peppers
- 1/4 cup of diced tomatoes
- 2 tablespoons of olive oil
- 2 tablespoons of freshly squeezed lime juice
- 1/2 teaspoon of ground cumin
- 1/4 teaspoon of salt

Instructions

1. Cook the quinoa according to the package instructions.

2. In a bowl, mix together the cooked quinoa, black beans, red onions, red bell peppers, and tomatoes.

3. Whisk together the olive oil, lime juice, cumin, and salt in a separate bowl.

4. Pour the dressing over the quinoa mixture and stir until everything is combined.

5. Serve the salad at room temperature.

Celery Sticks with Peanut Butter

Prep Time: 5 minutes   *Cook Time: 0 minutes*

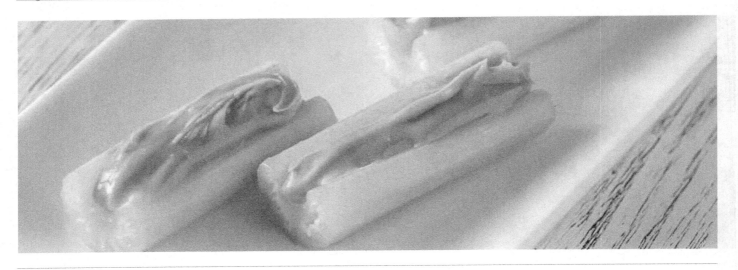

Ingredients

- 4 celery sticks
- 2 tablespoons of peanut butter

Instructions

1. Spread the peanut butter onto the celery sticks.
2. Serve the celery sticks at room temperature.

Salmon and Avocado Roll

Prep Time: 10 minutes

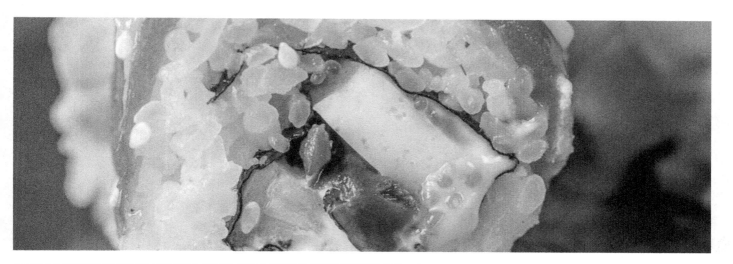

Ingredients

- 1 sheet of nori
- 1/4 cup cooked salmon
- 1/4 avocado, sliced
- 1/4 cup cooked sushi rice

Instructions

1. Lay a sheet of nori on a flat surface.
2. Place the cooked sushi rice onto the sheet of nori and spread it out evenly.
3. Place the cooked salmon and avocado slices onto the rice.
4. Roll the nori up tightly and slice it into eight pieces.
5. Serve with soy sauce and wasabi

Carrot Sticks with Tahini

Prep Time: 10 minutes

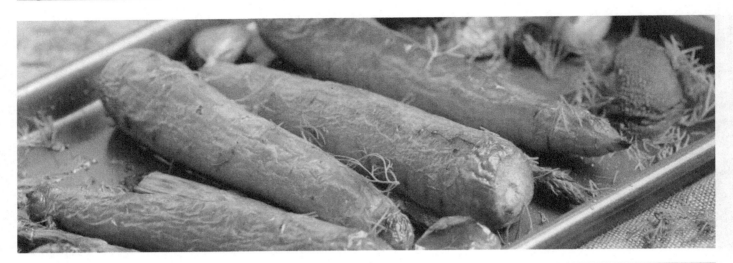

Ingredients

- 3 carrots, peeled and cut into sticks
- 2 tablespoons tahini
- 2 tablespoons lemon juice
- Salt and pepper, to taste

Instructions

1. Preheat oven to 375 degrees F.
2. Place the carrot sticks onto a baking sheet and bake for 15 minutes.
3. In a small bowl, mix together the tahini, lemon juice, salt, and pepper.
4. Serve the carrot sticks with the tahini dip on the side.

Seaweed Snack

Prep Time: 5 minutes

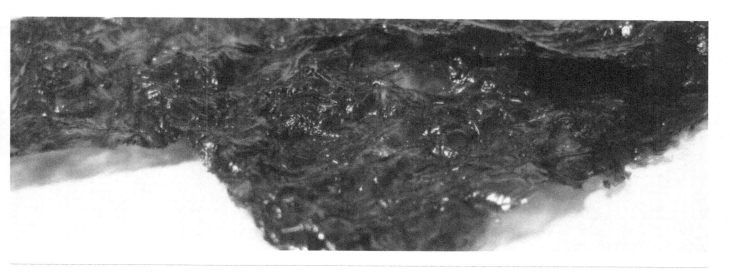

Ingredients

- 2 sheets of nori
- 2 tablespoons sesame seeds
- 2 tablespoons tamari

Instructions

1. Preheat oven to 350 degrees F.
2. Place the nori sheets onto a baking sheet.
3. Sprinkle the sesame seeds and tamari over the nori sheets.
4. Bake for 5 minutes or until crisp.
5. Serve as a snack.

Coconut Yogurt with Granola

Prep Time: 10 minutes

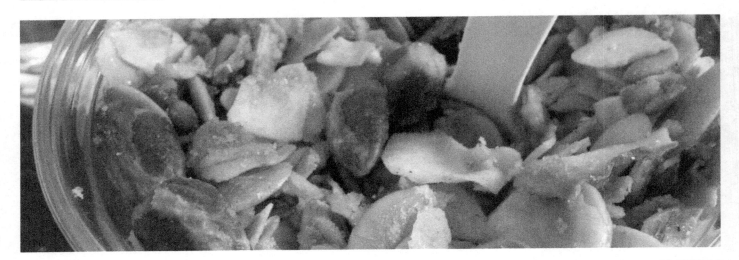

Ingredients

- 1 cup coconut yogurt
- 1/2 cup granola
- 1/4 cup fresh fruit (berries, banana, etc.)
- 1 tablespoon honey (optional)

Instructions

1. Place the coconut yogurt into a bowl.
2. Top with the granola, fresh fruit, and honey (if using).
3. Enjoy!

Dessert Recipes for the Mind Diet for Alzheimer's and Dementia

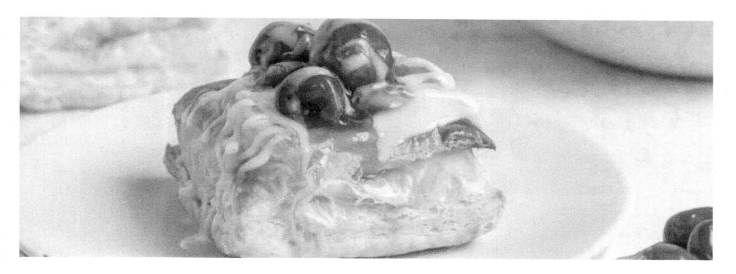

Desserts can be a part of the Mind Diet, and there are many delicious and healthy options available.

Some great dessert recipes for the Mind Diet include fruit-based desserts like fruit salads, baked apples, or fruit skewers

Banana Berry Smoothie

Prep Time: 5 minutes

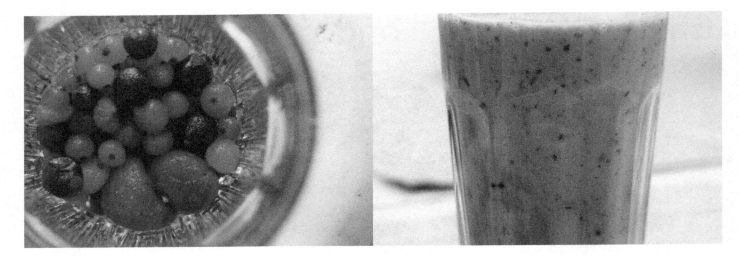

Ingredients

- 1 ripe banana
- ½ cup frozen blueberries
- ½ cup frozen raspberries
- 1 cup almond milk
- 1 teaspoon honey

Instructions

1. Place the banana, frozen berries, almond milk, and honey in a blender.
2. Blend on high speed until smooth.
3. Serve immediately.

Apple Cinnamon Muffins

Prep Time: 15 minutes

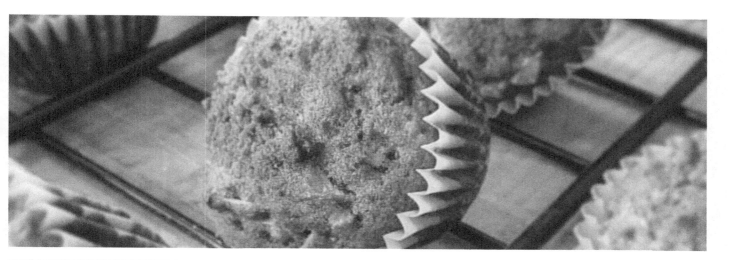

Ingredients

- 2 cups all-purpose flour
- 2 teaspoons baking powder
- 1 teaspoon ground cinnamon
- ½ teaspoon salt
- ⅓ cup melted butter
- ¾ cup brown sugar
- 2 large eggs
- 1 cup grated apple
- ½ cup chopped walnuts

Instructions

1. Preheat oven to 350°F. Grease with butter a 12-cup muffin tin or spray with cooking spray.

2. In a medium bowl, whisk together the flour, baking powder, cinnamon, and salt.

3. In a separate bowl, mix together the butter, brown sugar, and eggs until creamy.

4. Add the dry ingredients to the wet ingredients and mix until combined.

5. Fold in the grated apple and walnuts.

6. Divide the batter evenly among the muffin cups.

7. Bake for 18-20 minutes, or until a toothpick inserted in the center of a muffin comes out clean.

8. Let cool before serving

Avocado Mousse

Prep Time: 10 minutes

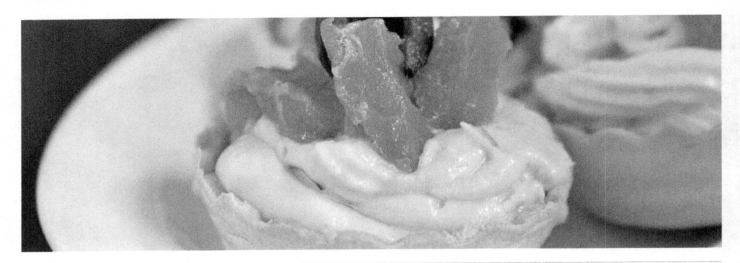

Ingredients

- 2 ripe avocados
- 2 tablespoons fresh lime juice
- ¼ cup honey
- ¼ cup coconut cream
- 1 teaspoon vanilla extract

Instructions

1. Place the avocados and lime juice in a food processor and blend until smooth.

2. Add the honey, coconut cream, and vanilla extract. Blend again until smooth.

3. Scoop the mousse into individual serving dishes.

4. Refrigerate for at least 1 hour before serving.

Baked Apple with Cinnamon and Honey

Prep Time: 15 minutes

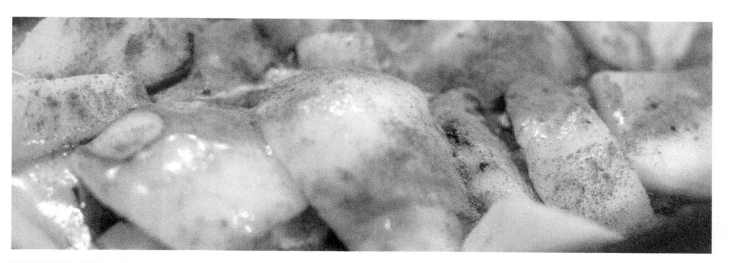

Ingredients

- 2 large apples
- 2 tablespoons butter
- 2 tablespoons brown sugar
- 2 tablespoons honey
- ½ teaspoon ground cinnamon

Instructions

1. Preheat oven to 350°F. Grease a baking dish with butter.
2. Core and slice the apples into ½-inch slices.
3. Place the apple slices in the baking dish.
4. In a small bowl, mix together the butter, brown sugar, honey, and cinnamon.
5. Spoon the mixture over the apples.
6. Bake for 20 minutes or until the apples are tender.
7. Serve warm.

Blueberry Coconut Quinoa Pudding

Prep Time: 15 minutes

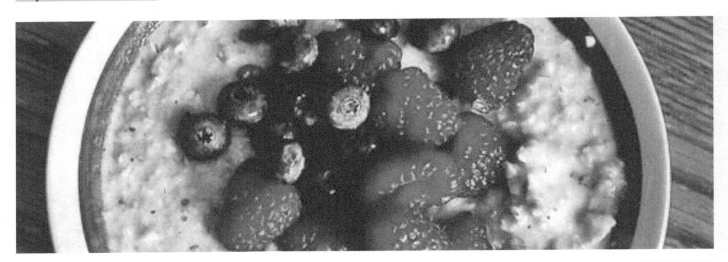

Ingredients

- 1 cup cooked quinoa
- ¾ cup coconut milk
- 2 tablespoons honey
- ¼ teaspoon ground cinnamon
- ½ cup fresh blueberries

Instructions

1. Place the cooked quinoa, coconut milk, honey, and cinnamon in a medium bowl. Stir until combined.

2. Divide the quinoa mixture into four serving dishes.

3. Top each dish with blueberries.

4. Refrigerate for at least 1 hour before serving.

Carrot Cake with Cream Cheese Frosting

Prep Time: 25 minutes

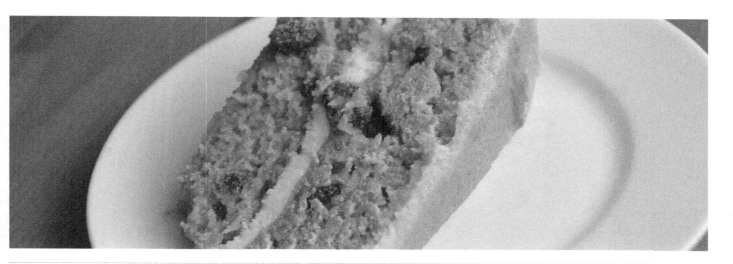

Ingredients

- 2 cups all-purpose flour
- 2 teaspoons baking powder
- 2 teaspoons ground cinnamon
- ½ teaspoon ground ginger
- ½ teaspoon salt
- 1 cup vegetable oil
- 1 cup sugar
- 2 large eggs
- 1 teaspoon vanilla extract
- 2 cups grated carrots
- 1 cup chopped walnuts
- 8 ounces cream cheese, softened
- ¼ cup butter, softened
- 2 cups powdered sugar

Instructions

1. Preheat oven to 350°F. Grease with butter a 9-inch round cake pan or spray with cooking spray.

2. In a medium bowl, whisk together the flour, baking powder, cinnamon, ginger, and salt.

3. In a separate bowl, mix together the oil, sugar, eggs, and vanilla extract until creamy.

4. Add the dry ingredients to the wet ingredients and mix until combined.

5. Fold in the grated carrots and walnuts.

6. Pour the batter into the prepared cake pan.

7. Bake for 25-30 minutes, or until a toothpick inserted in the center of the cake comes out clean.

8. Let cool before frosting.

9. To make the frosting, combine the cream cheese and butter in a medium bowl. Beat until creamy.

10. Add in the powdered sugar and mix until combined.

11. Spread the frosting over the cooled cake.

12. Serve immediately.

Chocolate Chia Pudding

Prep Time: 5 minutes

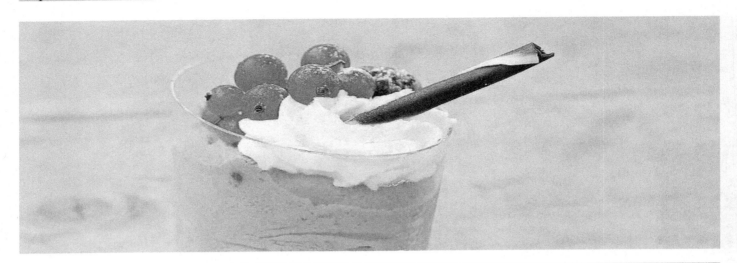

Ingredients

- ¼ cup chia seeds
- 1 cup almond milk
- 2 tablespoons cocoa powder
- 2 tablespoons honey

Instructions

1. Place the chia seeds, almond milk, cocoa powder, and honey in a medium bowl. Stir until combined.

2. Cover and refrigerate for at least 4 hours or overnight.

3. Serve chilled.

Coconut Yogurt Parfaits

Prep Time: 5 minutes

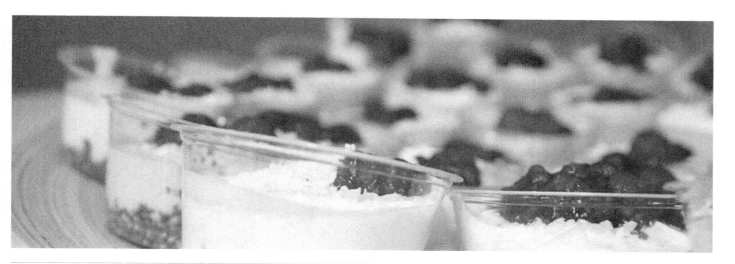

Ingredients

- 2 cups coconut yogurt
- 2 tablespoons honey
- ½ cup fresh blueberries
- ½ cup chopped almonds

Instructions

1. Place ½ cup of the yogurt in the bottom of four individual serving dishes.
2. Drizzle with one tablespoon of honey.
3. Top with ¼ cup of blueberries and ¼ cup of almonds.
4. Repeat layering with the remaining yogurt, honey, blueberries, and almonds.
5. Serve immediately.

Date Walnut Squares

Prep Time: 20 minutes

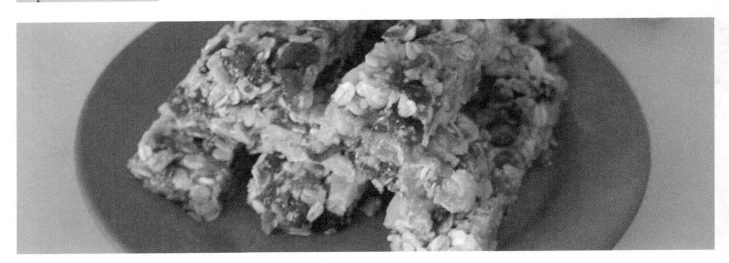

Ingredients

- 1 cup pitted dates
- ¾ cup chopped walnuts
- ¼ cup almond butter
- ¼ cup honey

Instructions

1. Preheat oven to 350°F. Grease an 8-inch square baking dish with butter or cooking spray.
2. Place the dates in a food processor and blend until smooth.
3. Add the walnuts, almond butter, and honey. Blend until combined.
4. Spread the mixture into the prepared baking dish.
5. Bake for 15 minutes or until golden brown.
6. Let cool before slicing into squares.

Fruit Salad with Lemon Poppy Seed Dressing

Prep Time: 15 minutes

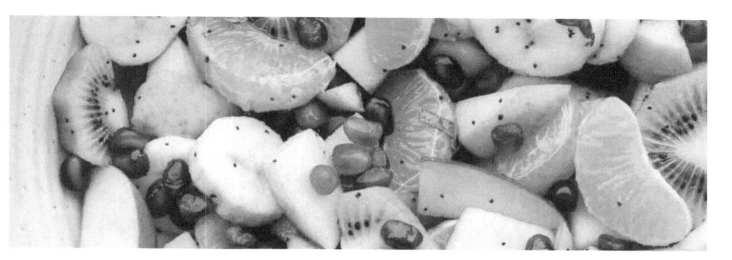

Ingredients

- 2 cups chopped fresh fruit (strawberries, blueberries, raspberries, apples, etc.)
- 2 tablespoons honey
- 2 tablespoons lemon juice
- ½ teaspoon poppy seeds

Instructions

1. Place the chopped fruit in a large bowl.
2. In a small bowl, whisk together the honey, lemon juice, and poppy seeds.
3. Pour the dressing over the fruit and gently toss to combine.
4. Refrigerate for at least 1 hour before serving.

Granola with Almonds and Raisins

Prep Time: 10 minutes   *Cook Time:* 20 minutes

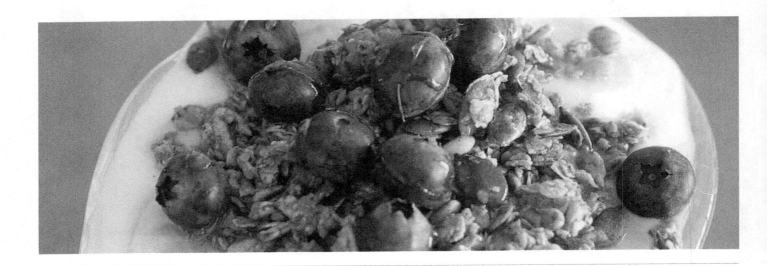

Ingredients

- 3 cups rolled oats
- 1 cup slivered almonds
- 1 cup raisins
- 1/2 cup packed brown sugar
- 1/2 teaspoon ground cinnamon
- 1/4 teaspoon ground nutmeg
- 1/2 cup vegetable oil
- 1/3 cup honey

Instructions

1. Preheat oven to 350°F.

2. In a large bowl, combine oats, almonds, raisins, brown sugar, cinnamon, and nutmeg.

3. In a separate bowl, whisk together oil and honey.

4. Pour the oil and honey mixture over the oat mixture and stir until everything is well combined.

5. Spread the mixture onto a greased baking sheet.

6. Bake for 20 minutes, stirring halfway through.

7. Let cool before serving.

Greek Yogurt Popsicles

Prep Time: 10 minutes *Freezing Time: 6 hours*

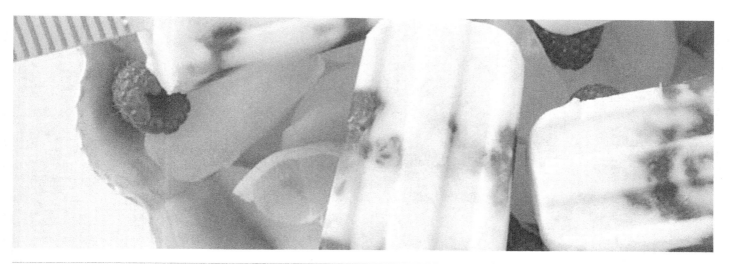

Ingredients

- 2 cups Greek yogurt
- 1/2 cup honey
- 1/2 teaspoon vanilla extract
- 1/2 teaspoon ground cinnamon
- 1/4 cup chopped almonds

Instructions

1. Whisk together the yogurt, honey, vanilla extract, and cinnamon in a medium bowl.

2. Pour the mixture into popsicle molds, then top with chopped almonds.

3. Place the popsicles in the freezer and freeze for 6 hours or until solid.

4. Once frozen, remove from the molds and enjoy.

Honeydew Melon with Mint

Prep Time: 10 minutes

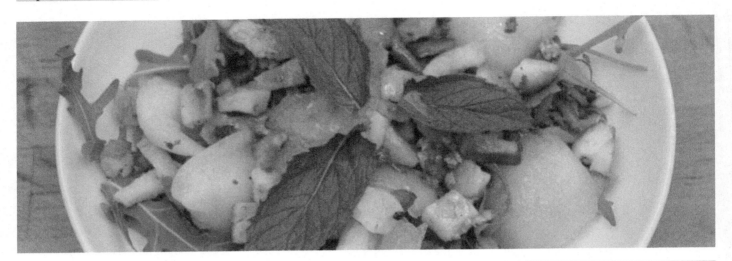

Ingredients

- 1 honeydew melon, cut into cubes
- 1/4 cup fresh mint leaves
- 2 tablespoons honey

Instructions

1. Place the honeydew melon cubes in a large bowl.
2. Add the mint leaves and honey and toss to combine.
3. Serve chilled.

Lemon Poppy Seed Bars

Prep Time: 10 minutes   *Cook Time: 25 minutes*

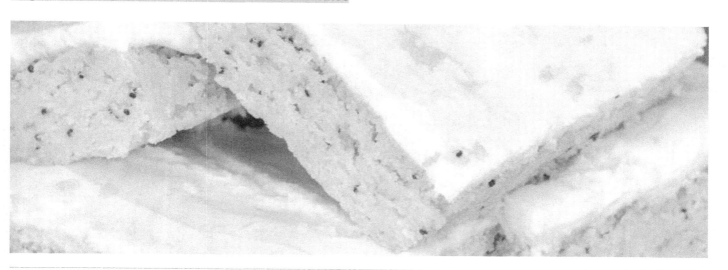

Ingredients

- 1 cup all-purpose flour
- 1/2 cup granulated sugar
- 1/2 teaspoon baking powder
- 1/2 teaspoon salt
- 2 tablespoons poppy seeds
- 1/2 cup butter, melted
- 2 large eggs
- 1/4 cup fresh lemon juice
- 1 teaspoon lemon zest

Instructions

1. Preheat oven to 350°F.
2. Grease an 8x8-inch baking pan.
3. Whisk together the flour, sugar, baking powder, salt, and poppy seeds in large bowl.
4. In a separate bowl, whisk together the melted butter, eggs, lemon juice, and lemon zest.
5. Pour the wet ingredients into the dry ingredients and stir until combined.
6. Pour the mixture into the prepared pan and spread evenly.
7. Bake for 25 minutes, or until a toothpick inserted into the center comes out clean.
8. Let cool before serving.

Oatmeal Raisin Cookies

Prep Time: 15 minutes   *Cook Time: 10 minutes*

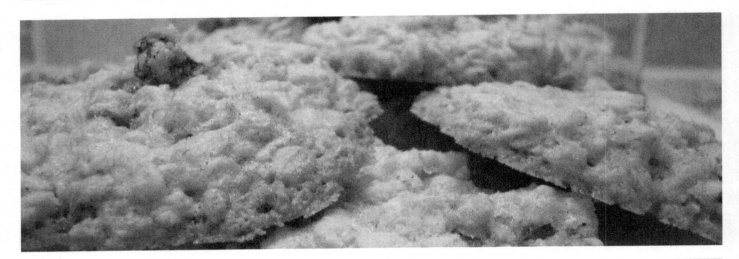

Ingredients

- 1 cup all-purpose flour
- 1/2 cup granulated sugar
- 1/2 teaspoon baking powder
- 1/2 teaspoon salt
- 2 tablespoons poppy seeds
- 1/2 cup butter, melted
- 2 large eggs
- 1/4 cup fresh lemon juice
- 1 teaspoon lemon zest

Instructions

1. Preheat oven to 350°F.
2. Grease an 8x8-inch baking pan.
3. Whisk together the flour, sugar, baking powder, salt, and poppy seeds in large bowl.
4. In a separate bowl, whisk together the melted butter, eggs, lemon juice, and lemon zest.
5. Pour the wet ingredients into the dry ingredients and stir until combined.
6. Pour the mixture into the prepared pan and spread evenly.
7. Bake for 25 minutes, or until a toothpick inserted into the center comes out clean.
8. Let cool before serving.

Peach Cobbler

Prep Time: 10 minutes   *Cook Time: 40 minutes*

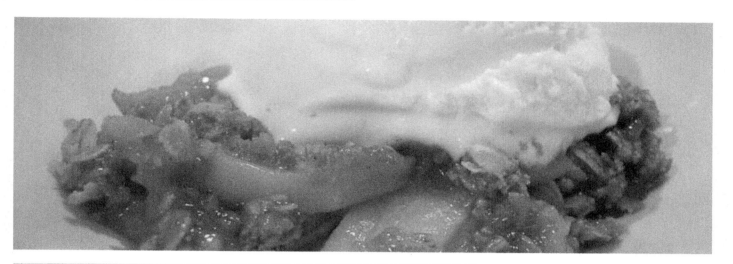

Ingredients

- 4 cups peeled, sliced peaches
- 1/2 cup granulated sugar
- 1 teaspoon ground cinnamon
- 1/2 teaspoon ground nutmeg
- 1/2 cup all-purpose flour
- 1/2 cup packed brown sugar
- 1/2 cup butter, melted

Instructions

1. Preheat oven to 375°F.
2. Place the peaches in an 8x8-inch baking dish.
3. In a medium bowl, combine the granulated sugar, cinnamon, and nutmeg.
4. Sprinkle the sugar mixture over the peaches and stir until combined.
5. In a separate bowl, whisk together the flour and brown sugar.
6. Pour the melted butter over the flour mixture and stir until combined.
7. Crumble the mixture over the peaches.
8. Bake for 40 minutes or until golden brown.
9. Let cool before serving.

Pear Crumble

Prep Time: 10 minutes *Cook Time: 40 minutes*

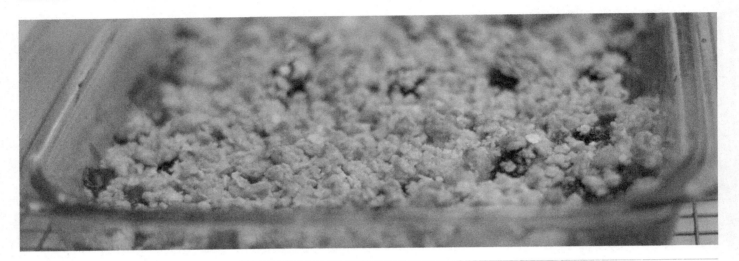

Ingredients

- 4 cups peeled, sliced pears
- 1/2 cup granulated sugar
- 1 teaspoon ground cinnamon
- 1/2 teaspoon ground nutmeg
- 1/2 cup all-purpose flour
- 1/2 cup packed brown sugar
- 1/2 cup butter, melted

Instructions

1. Preheat oven to 375°F.
2. Place the pears in an 8x8-inch baking dish.
3. In a medium bowl, combine the granulated sugar, cinnamon, and nutmeg.
4. Sprinkle the sugar mixture over the pears and stir until combined.
5. In a separate bowl, whisk together the flour and brown sugar.
6. Pour the melted butter over the flour mixture and stir until combined.
7. Crumble the mixture over the pears.
8. Bake for 40 minutes or until golden brown.
9. Let cool before serving

Pineapple and Coconut Custard

Prep Time: 10 minutes   *Cook Time: 30 minutes*

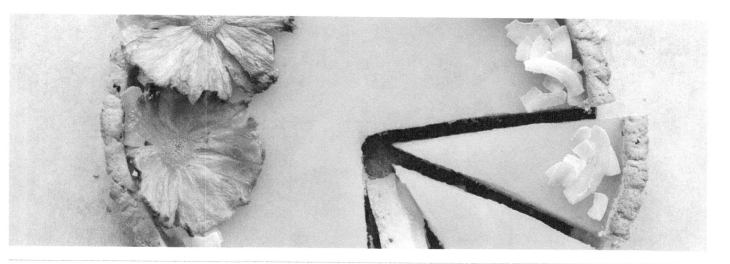

Ingredients

- 1 cup pineapple, chopped
- 1/2 cup coconut milk
- 1/4 cup granulated sugar
- 2 large eggs
- 1 teaspoon vanilla extract

Instructions

1. Preheat oven to 350°F.
2. Grease a 9-inch baking dish.
3. Place the pineapple in the baking dish.
4. In a medium bowl, whisk together the coconut milk, sugar, eggs, and vanilla extract.
5. Pour the mixture over the pineapple.
6. Bake for 30 minutes or until set.
7. Let cool before serving.

Roasted Plums with Ricotta

Prep Time: 10 minutes   *Cook Time: 20 minutes*

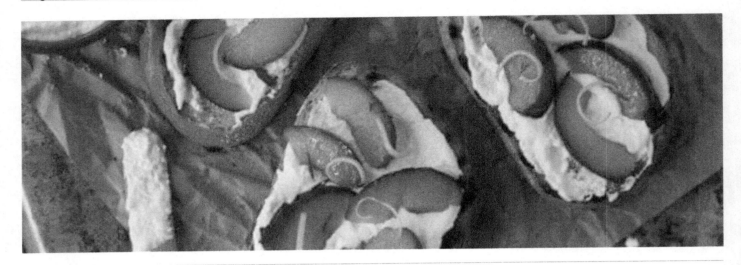

Ingredients

- 4 plums, halved and pitted
- 1/4 cup honey
- 1/4 teaspoon ground cinnamon
- 1/4 teaspoon ground nutmeg
- 1/2 cup ricotta cheese

Instructions

1. Preheat oven to 400°F.
2. Place the plums on a baking sheet and drizzle with honey.
3. Sprinkle with cinnamon and nutmeg.
4. Roast for 20 minutes or until tender.
5. Top with ricotta cheese and serve.

Sliced Strawberries with Balsamic Glaze

Prep Time: 10 minutes   *Cook Time: 10 minutes*

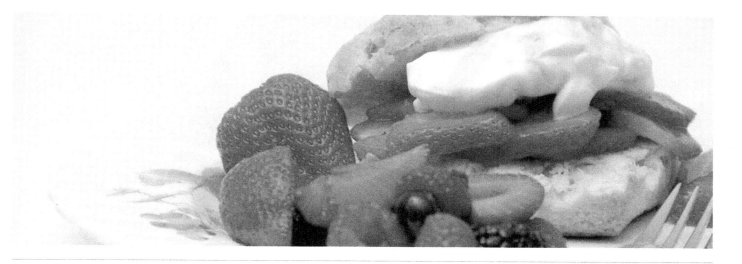

Ingredients

- 2 cups sliced strawberries
- 1/2 cup balsamic vinegar
- 2 tablespoons honey

Instructions

1. Place the sliced strawberries in a bowl.
2. In a small saucepan, bring the balsamic vinegar to a boil over medium-high heat.
3. Reduce the heat to low and simmer for 10 minutes or until reduced by half.
4. Remove from heat and stir in the honey.
5. Drizzle the balsamic glaze over the strawberries and serve.

Spiced Apple Cake

Prep Time: 15 minutes   *Cook Time: 60 minutes*   *Serves: 12*

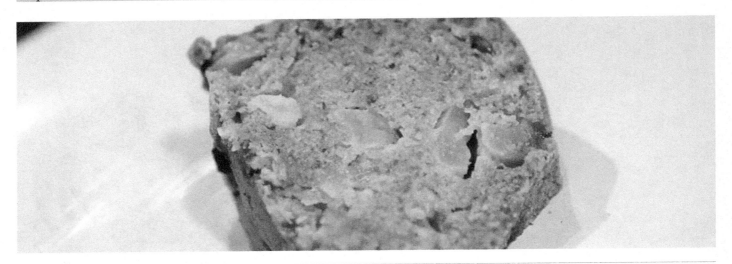

Ingredients

- 2 teaspoons baking powder
- 1 teaspoon ground cinnamon
- ½ teaspoon ground nutmeg
- ½ teaspoon ground ginger
- ¼ teaspoon ground allspice
- ¼ teaspoon ground cloves
- ½ teaspoon salt
- 1 cup unsalted butter, softened
- 1¾ cups packed light brown sugar
- 4 large eggs
- ¾ cup whole milk
- 2 teaspoons pure vanilla extract
- 4 large apples, peeled, cored, and diced

Instructions

1. Preheat oven to 350°F. Grease and flour a 9x13-inch baking pan.

2. Whisk together flour, baking powder, cinnamon, nutmeg, ginger, allspice, cloves, and salt in a medium bowl.

3. In a large bowl, using an electric mixer, beat together butter and brown sugar until light and fluffy. Break in the eggs one at a time, followed by the milk and vanilla.

4. Slowly add in flour mixture and beat until just combined. Stir in diced apples.

5. Pour batter into the prepared pan and spread evenly. Bake for 60 minutes, until a toothpick inserted into the center, comes out clean. Before cutting and serving, allow cooling completely on a wire rack.

Strawberry Cream Cheese Pie

Prep Time: 10 minutes   *Cook Time: 30 minutes*   *Serves: 8*

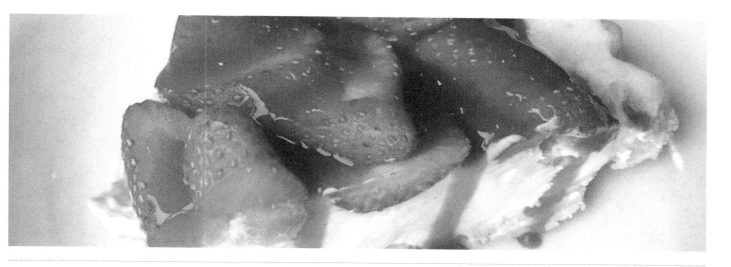

Ingredients

- 1 store-bought graham cracker crust
- 8 ounces cream cheese, softened
- ¼ cup granulated sugar
- ½ teaspoon pure vanilla extract
- 2 cups fresh strawberries, hulled and sliced
- 2 tablespoons strawberry jam
- 1 cup heavy cream, chilled
- 2 tablespoons confectioners' sugar

Instructions

1. Preheat oven to 350°F.

2. In a large bowl, using an electric mixer, beat cream cheese, sugar, and vanilla until light and fluffy.

3. Spread the cream cheese mixture into the prepared graham cracker crust and spread evenly. Top with sliced strawberries.

4. Bake for 30 minutes, until edges are lightly golden brown. Cool completely on a wire rack.

5. In a medium bowl, beat together strawberry jam and heavy cream until soft peaks form. Gradually add in confectioners' sugar, beating until stiff peaks form.

6. Spread strawberry whipped cream over cooled pie and chill until ready to serve.

Trail Mix Bites

Prep Time: 10 minutes *Cook Time: 25 minutes* *Serves: 24 bites*

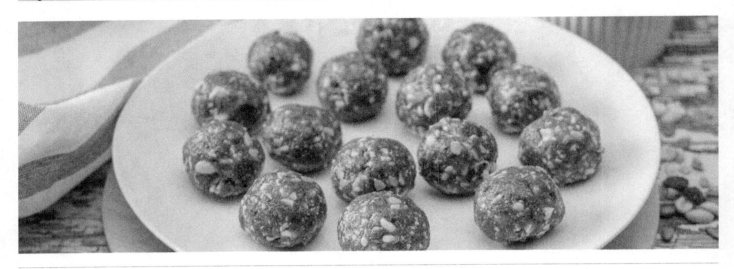

Ingredients

- 2 cups old-fashioned rolled oats
- ¼ cup honey
- ¼ cup peanut butter
- 1 teaspoon ground cinnamon
- ½ teaspoon pure vanilla extract
- ¼ teaspoon salt
- ½ cup chopped walnuts
- ½ cup dried cranberries
- ½ cup dark chocolate chips

Instructions

1. Preheat oven to 350°F. Line a baking sheet with parchment paper.

2. In a large bowl, stir together oats, honey, peanut butter, cinnamon, vanilla, and salt until well combined. Stir in walnuts, cranberries, and chocolate chips.

3. Using a small cookie scoop, scoop the mixture onto the prepared baking sheet, spacing them about 2 inches apart. Bake for 25 minutes, until golden brown. Cool completely on a wire rack.

Vanilla Yogurt with Fresh Fruit

Prep Time: 5 minutes   *Serves: 1*

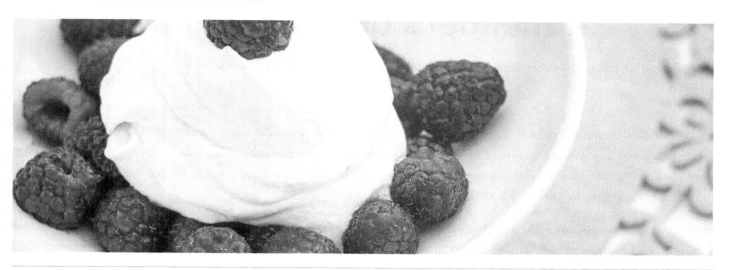

Ingredients

- ½ cup plain Greek yogurt
- 1 teaspoon pure vanilla extract
- 1 tablespoon honey
- ½ cup fresh fruit (strawberries, blueberries, bananas, etc.)

Instructions

1. In a small bowl, stir together yogurt, vanilla, and honey until well combined.
2. Spoon the yogurt mixture into a bowl and top with fresh fruit. Serve immediately.

More Approaches to Managing Alzheimer's and Dementia

In this section, we will explore more approaches to managing Alzheimer's and Dementia.

A. Exercise

Exercise can be a powerful tool in managing Alzheimer's and dementia. Physical activity can help slow the progression of these diseases and improve the quality of life for those affected. Exercise increases blood flow to the brain and helps with mental stimulation, as well as improving mood and overall physical health. It can also aid to reduce the risk of falls, which is particularly important for those with Alzheimer's and dementia.

Regular exercise can help strengthen the body and improve balance, coordination, and flexibility. This can help reduce the risk of falls and injuries, which can be particularly dangerous for those with Alzheimer's and dementia. Exercise also increases cardiovascular health, which can help with brain health. Regular physical activity can help improve cognitive function and reduce the risk of memory loss and confusion.

Exercise can also help with mood and mental health. Physical activity can help increase endorphins, which can help reduce stress and anxiety. Exercise can also help those with Alzheimer's and dementia stay socially active and engaged. This can enhance their general wellbeing and lessen feelings of isolation and loneliness.

It is important to remember that Alzheimer's and dementia can affect everyone differently, so it is important to talk to a doctor to determine the best type of exercise for each individual. It is important to start slowly and gradually increase the amount of activity over time. Exercise should be tailored to the individual's level of ability and should be fun and enjoyable.

Exercise can be a powerful tool in managing Alzheimer's and dementia and can help improve the overall quality of life. It is important to speak to a doctor before starting any exercise program, but with the right guidance, exercise can be a valuable part of a healthy lifestyle for those affected by these diseases.

B. Stress Management

Stress management is an important part of a holistic approach to supporting people living with Alzheimer's and other forms of dementia. Stress can significantly affect people's lives of people living with dementia and their caregivers. It can worsen symptoms, interfere with managing the disease, and reduce the quality of life for both the person living with dementia and their caregivers.

There are several ways to manage stress for people living with dementia and their caregivers. Regular physical activity, relaxation techniques, and meaningful activities can all help reduce stress. It is important to provide a supportive environment that promotes physical and emotional well-being.

Regular physical activity can help reduce stress and improve overall health. Exercise can help improve physical functioning, psychological well-being, and cognitive functioning. It can also reduce stress and anxiety and improve mood. Regular physical activities have been shown to be beneficial for people living with dementia, and it can help caregivers too.

Relaxation techniques, such as deep breathing, muscle relaxation, and mindfulness, can help reduce stress and improve overall well-being. Relaxation can help reduce anxiety, improve mood, and increase feelings of calmness.

Meaningful activities can also provide an outlet for stress. Activities that involve physical movement, such as dancing or gardening, can provide physical and mental stimulation. Social activities, such as visiting family, going to a movie, or attending a support group, can help reduce feelings of isolation and provide a sense of belonging.

Stress management is an important part of caring for someone living with dementia. It can aid to improve the quality of life for both the person living with dementia and their caregivers. Regular physical activity, relaxation techniques, and meaningful activities can all help reduce stress and improve overall health.

C. Social Connections

Social connections can play an important part in helping to manage Alzheimer's and Dementia for both the person with the condition and their family. Social connections can provide a sense of community and support, help to maintain a sense of identity, provide opportunities to stay engaged in meaningful activities and provide stimulation that can help to slow the progression of the condition.

For individuals with Alzheimer's or Dementia, social connections can help to maintain their sense of identity and self-worth, provide an outlet for emotions, and reduce feelings of isolation and loneliness. Building and maintaining social connections with family, friends, and the community can give the individual something to look forward to and keep them engaged in meaningful activities. This can also provide an opportunity to learn new skills and stay connected to their community.

For family and caregivers, having a support network of family and friends is essential. It can provide emotional support, help with practical tasks related to caregiving, and give the caregiver a chance to take regular breaks. Social connections can also help to reduce stress and provide resources that can help the family and caregiver to better understand and manage the condition.

Social connections can also help to slow the progression of Alzheimer's and Dementia. By engaging in activities and meaningful conversations, the individual can continue to use their existing skills and learn new ones. This can help to maintain cognitive functioning and delay the onset of more severe symptoms.

Overall, social connections can play an important role in helping to manage Alzheimer's and Dementia. They can provide support, reduce stress, and help to maintain a sense of identity and self-worth. They can also provide an opportunity to learn and stay engaged in meaningful activities, helping to slow the progression of the condition.

Conclusion

The Complete Mind Diet Cookbook for Beginners is an excellent resource for people living with Alzheimer's and dementia. The cookbook provides an easy-to-follow guide to the Msssssind Diet, outlining the key principles and providing a variety of delicious recipes to enjoy. Eating mindfully and healthily can improve physical and mental health, and this cookbook provides recipes that are tailored to the needs of those living with Alzheimer's and dementia. The recipes are simple, nutritious, and creative and include plenty of fresh ingredients and superfoods that provide essential vitamins and minerals. With the help of this cookbook, people living with Alzheimer's and dementia can discover how to nourish their bodies, boost their moods, and sharpen their minds.

This cookbook is also for people willing to improve their physical and mental health. The recipes are designed for those who are short on time but still want to eat well. The cookbook also provides tips on shopping, meal planning, and nutrition. With this easy-to-follow guide, anyone can learn to nourish their bodies and minds with nutritious and delicious recipes.

The Complete Mind Diet Cookbook for Beginners is a must-have resource for anyone looking to improve their physical and mental health. The recipes are simple, nutritious, and creative, and they provide essential vitamins and minerals. With this cookbook, anyone can learn how to feed their bodies and minds with delicious and healthy meals.

Made in the USA
Monee, IL
30 May 2024

59100897R00090